The Thames Valley

The Chilterns and Oxford

by
F. R. BANKS

Letts Motor Tour Guides

Printed and Published by
Charles Letts & Company Limited
London, Edinburgh & New York

Head Office:
Diary House, Borough Road, London, S.E.1

Publishing Consultant: Lionel Leventhal

Cover Artist: Kenneth Farnhill

Maps: Jack Parker

The Thames Valley
by F. R. Banks
first published 1969
© Charles Letts & Company Limited, 1969

How to use your
Letts Motor Tour Guide

The best way to see Britain is, for most people, by car. This Tour Guide has been specially designed to lead you—the motorist—to all that is best in its chosen area.

The Thames Valley, Oxford and the Chiltern Hills

This series of tours explores a region well-loved by Londoners, the Thames Valley upstream to Oxford and the long chalk range of the Chiltern Hills, but it also includes the Vale of Aylesbury and other quiet and little-known country beyond the Chilterns, as well as the valleys of the Great Ouse and the Lea.

The Tours

There are ten motor tours in this guide and each tour covers less than a hundred miles. If you wish to visit and explore all the places mentioned, you may find that a single tour will provide two or more good days' motoring. All the tours are circular, and so you can start and finish a route at any other point you may choose. The book is yours to use in your own way.

The Maps

The maps (one for each tour and a larger one for the whole area) have been specially designed to show clearly all the information you will need—without being unduly technical. Readers who lack expertise in map-reading will have no difficulty in following the directions and the route. The main approach roads to the tours are also indicated.

Reference Books

For those who wish to use more detailed maps, Sheet 17 of the Ordnance Survey quarter-inch maps covers most of the area, while Sheets 16 and 13 take in the western and northern fringes.

Particulars are given in the tours of the days and times of opening for houses, castles and museums, and these are correct at the time

of going to press. The most recent information can be obtained from *Historic Houses, Castles and Gardens in Great Britain,* which is published annually in February. Details regarding museums and art galleries are given in *Museums and Galleries in Great Britain,* published yearly in July.

Particulars of hotels, restaurants and inns are given in the annual reference guide, *Hotels and Restaurants in Britain,* published by the British Travel Association. An annual selective and critical guide to eating places is Raymond Postgate's *Good Food Guide,* and a more extensive annual critical guide to hotels, restaurants, pubs and inns is written by Egon Ronay. All the above books may be purchased from any bookseller, or referred to at a library.

This Series

This Motor Tour Guide is part of a continuing series which will cover the whole of the British Isles. Every effort has been made to ensure the accuracy at the time of going to press of all factual information, but some of this is of the kind which may change from year to year. The publishers would therefore be grateful if readers would draw their attention to any improvements which may be made to these Motor Tour Guides. In this way, future editions can be made as complete and useful as possible. Other titles in this series are:

Devon and Cornwall by Wilfrid E. Rolfe

Kent, Surrey and Sussex by Bryant Peers

Stratford and the Cotswolds by Wilfrid E. Rolfe

The Lake District by F. R. Banks

The Highlands by F. R. Banks

Somerset and Dorset by Wilfrid E. Rolfe

The Peak District by F. R. Banks

North Wales and Anglesey by J. H. B. Peel

The North-West Highlands and Skye by F. R. Banks

LONDON BOROUGH OF LEWISHAM

LIBRARIES DEPARTMENT

Books must be returned on or before the last date stamped below or on the date card. Fines on overdue books will be charged:— $\frac{1}{2}$d per day for the first week (1d minimum), 1d per day for the second week. 2d per day thereafter.

Books are renewable by phone, letter or personal call unless required by another reader.

ALL LIBRARIES are closed on Sundays, Good Friday, Christmas Day, Bank Holidays, and the Saturdays prior to Bank Holidays.

Contents

Maps

Tour Maps are on the first or second page of each tour.

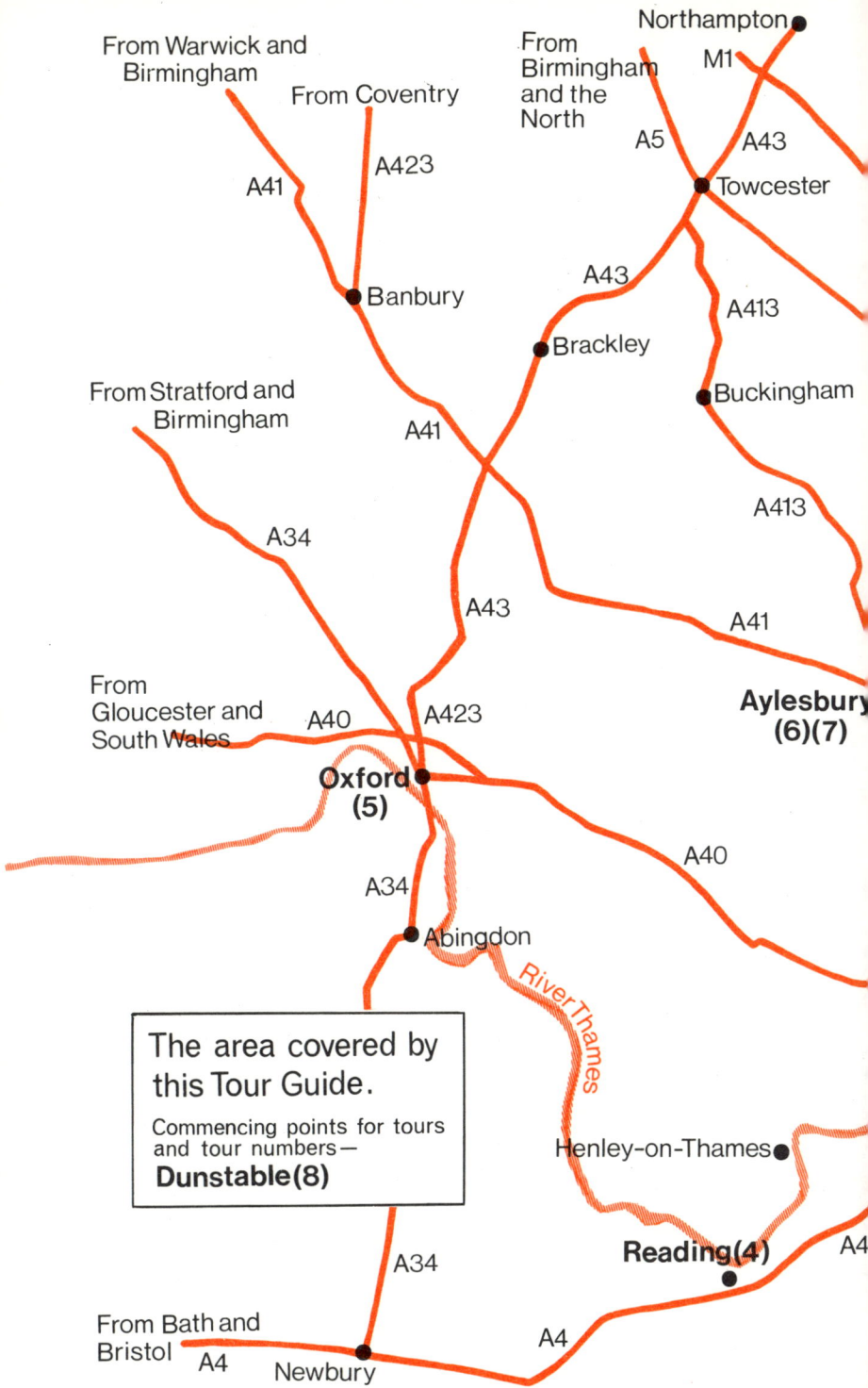

From Warwick and Birmingham

From Coventry

A41

A423

From Birmingham and the North

Northampton

M1

A5

A43

Towcester

Banbury

A43

Brackley

A413

Buckingham

From Stratford and Birmingham

A41

A413

A34

A43

A41

From Gloucester and South Wales

A40

A423

Aylesbury (6)(7)

Oxford (5)

A40

A34

Abingdon

River Thames

The area covered by this Tour Guide.

Commencing points for tours and tour numbers—
Dunstable(8)

Henley-on-Thames

Reading(4)

A4

A34

A4

From Bath and Bristol

A4

Newbury

A4

From Leicester,
Derby and Manchester

From Stamford and
the North

A1

A6

● Bedford

● Newport Pagnell

M1

A5

A6

M1

Dunstable
(8)

● Luton

A1

● Welwyn

From
Cambridge

A6

A41

A10

Hemel
Hempstead ●

A5

St.
Albans

● Hertford

A413

M1

A6

A41

A5

A10

Amersham ●

Watford ●

High Wycombe ●

Rickmansworth

M1

A41

A406

Hendon ●

A1

Harrow ●

A41

London
(1)(9)(10)

A40

A406

A5

Maidenhead ●

A4

Slough

A406

Marble Arch ●

M4

A4

Hyde Park
Corner

A332

M4

A4

Chiswick

A3

River
Thames

Windsor
(2)(3)

London
Airport

A4

Richmond ●

A308

A307

Staines

Kingston ●

A3

From
Salisbury
and Exeter

Chertsey ●

Esher ●

A3

From Portsmouth

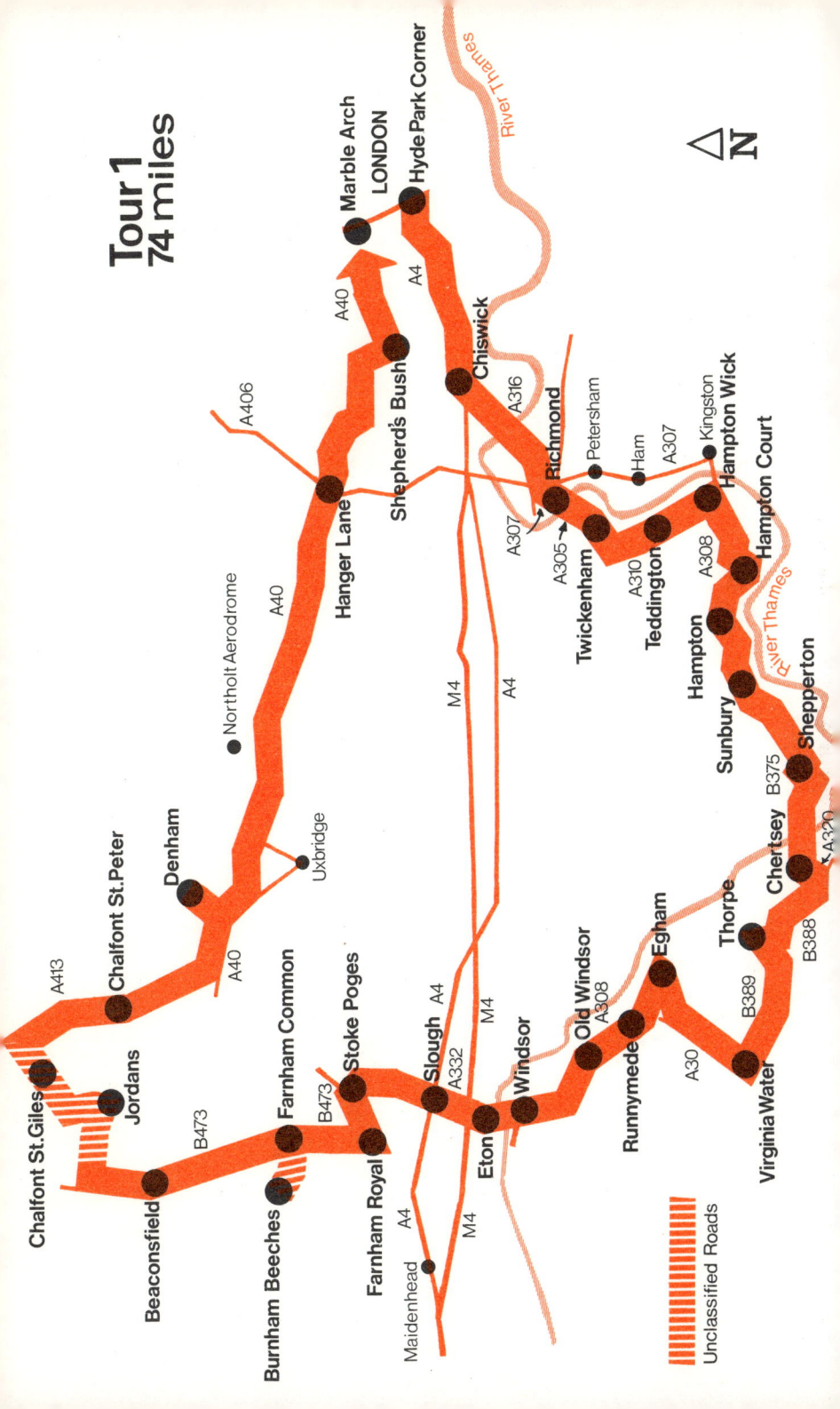

Tour 1
74 miles

N

Marble Arch
LONDON
Hyde Park Corner

River Thames

A40

A4

Shepherd's Bush

Chiswick

A316

A406

A307

Richmond

Petersham

Ham

A307

Hanger Lane

A305

Twickenham

Kingston

Hampton Wick

A40

A310

Teddington

Hampton Court

Northolt Aerodrome

A308

Hampton

River Thames

Sunbury

Shepperton

B375

Denham

Chalfont St.Peter

Uxbridge

Chertsey

B320

A413

Jordans

Thorpe

Farnham Common

B473

Stoke Poges

Slough

A4

Old Windsor

Egham

B389

B388

Virginia Water

Chalfont St.Giles

B473

B473

Farnham Royal

A332

Eton

Windsor

A308

Runnymede

A30

Beaconsfield

Burnham Beeches

M4

A4

M4

Maidenhead

M4

A4

Unclassified Roads

1. The Thames from London to Hampton Court and Windsor

The first four tours in this guide explore the Thames Valley from London as far upstream as Oxford. (The Thames above Oxford is described in another Letts Motor Tour Guide, *Stratford and the Cotswolds*). This first tour takes in the delightful old town of Richmond, and the magnificent royal palace of Hampton Court. It runs through Thameside villages to the old towns of Chertsey and Egham, then crosses the historic field of Runnymede on its way to Windsor, with its royal castle. The tour crosses the Thames to Eton, a pleasant small town famous for its college, and goes on via Stoke Poges, with its ' country churchyard,' Burnham Beeches, a lovely tract of old forest (best seen in the autumn), and Jordans, noted for its Quaker associations, and then returns down the valley of the Misbourne, passing the charming village of Denham.

From London (Hyde Park Corner) via Knightsbridge, Brompton Road, Cromwell Road and A4 to Hammersmith (flyover: 3 miles) and thence to Chiswick (roundabout: $1\frac{1}{2}$ miles more). A316 (Great Chertsey Road), crossing the Thames by Chiswick Bridge to Mortlake ($1\frac{1}{2}$ miles) and thence to North Sheen, then A307 (left) to Richmond (2 miles farther).

Richmond is a greatly favoured residential town delightfully placed on the slopes of a hill rising boldly from the Thames. Long associated with royalty, it became a resort of society during the 18th and early 19th centuries, and many fine mansions of this time have survived. The manor house of Sheen, converted into a palace by Edward III (who died here in 1377), was newly built by Henry VII, who changed its name to Richmond, after the title of his earldom derived from Richmond in Yorkshire. The king died in the palace in 1509 and Elizabeth I, who had been confined here during the reign of her sister Mary, also died here, in 1603. All that now remains are the brick gatehouse of about 1500 and an adjoining range of building, to the west of Richmond Green, which lies north of George Street, the main shopping street of Richmond. Bordering the green are charming 17th and 18th century terraces, including Maids of Honour Row, built about 1724 for the ladies-in-waiting to Princess Caroline of Anspach. George Street is continued south by Hill Street to the approach to the graceful Richmond Bridge, built in 1777, and Hill Rise leads up to Richmond Hill, one of the most famous streets in England, with many 18th century residences. It ascends past the Terrace, a favourite promenade commanding a noble prospect up to the Thames as far as Windsor Castle, with the North Downs away to the left. In the foreground are the charming Terrace Gardens, stretching down towards the river, and the 17th century Ham House is seen among the trees. At the top of the hill is the entrance to Richmond Park, over 8 miles round and the most beautiful open space within easy reach of central

9

London. First enclosed by Charles I in 1637 as a hunting ground, it remains largely in its natural state, with herds of deer (to be treated with caution in May-July and October).

A305, crossing Richmond Bridge and passing through Twickenham ($\frac{1}{2}$ mile) by Richmond Road, then A310 (in about $\frac{1}{2}$ mile more) to Teddington (about $1\frac{1}{2}$ miles farther) and thence to Hampton Wick ($1\frac{1}{2}$ miles), opposite Kingston.

Twickenham is a mainly residential district bordering the Thames. Marble Hill House (admission Tuesday-Saturday and Bank Holiday Mondays 10 to 6 or dusk, Sundays from 2), in a public park on the left of Richmond Road, is a Palladian-style house built in 1728 for George II. Montpelier Row and Sion Row, to the west, are unspoilt terraces of the early 18th century, and between them is the fine Octagon Room, the only surviving part of Orleans House, built by James Gibbs in 1730 for Queen Caroline. York House (now the Town Hall of the Borough of Richmond), farther on, was the summer home from 1660 of the historian Earl of Clarendon. Strawberry Hill, to the right of the road before reaching Teddington, and now a Roman Catholic training college, is the famous Gothic Revival villa built for Horace Walpole, the author, who died here in 1797.

A308 from Hampton Wick, skirting Hampton Court Park and passing the south end of the triple avenue in Bushy Park, to Hampton Court ($1\frac{1}{2}$ miles).

Hampton Court is a village with a large green and several 17th-18th century houses, on the Thames at the gates of Hampton Court Palace (admission 9.30 to 4, 5 or 6; Sundays 2 to 4 or 5, in May-September 11 to 6). Surrounded by delightful gardens, in a large park bordered by the river, this is a fascinating mansion begun in 1514 by Thomas Wolsey, Archbishop of York and later Cardinal, and enlarged and enriched by Henry VIII after 1529, when Wolsey was obliged to present it to the king. The palace became the principal country seat of royalty and Edward VI was born here in 1537. On the accession of William III, in 1688, Sir Christopher Wren was commissioned to enlarge and improve the palace, but after the death of George II in 1760, it was never occupied by a reigning sovereign. The Great Gatehouse, altered for Henry VIII and again in 1773, admits to the Base Court, an excellent example of Tudor brickwork. Beyond is the Clock Court, the main courtyard of Wolsey's palace, named from the splendid astronomical clock made in 1540 for Henry VIII, on the face of Anne Boleyn's Gateway. The State Apartments, in the wings added by Wren, have ceilings painted by Antonio Verrio and other artists, and contain 16th-17th century tapestries and fine furniture, but are most famous for their paintings, mainly of the Italian schools. The Chapel Royal, built by Wolsey but enriched by Henry VIII, has a sumptuous timber ceiling, and the Great Hall, 106 feet long, built for the king, has a magnificent hammerbeam roof. The Great

Fountain Gardens, facing the principal facade of the palace, was laid out for William III. On the south of the palace are the Tudor Gardens, the Great Vine, planted in 1768 and noted for its black grapes, and the Lower Orangery, housing the famous 15th-century tempera cartoons of the Triumphs of Caesar by Andrea Mantegna; on the north are the Royal Tennis Court, built for Henry VIII, himself an enthusiastic player, and the celebrated Maze.

A308 on the north bank of the Thames to Hampton (1 mile).

Hampton is a pleasant residential village, with old cottages. Garrick's Villa (formerly Hampton House) was bought in 1754 by David Garrick, the actor, and altered for him by Robert Adam.

B375 (left) to Sunbury-on-Thames ($2\frac{1}{2}$ miles).

Sunbury is a residential district with an attractive village street. Sunbury Court, a house of about 1770, near the east end, is now a Salvation Army youth centre.

B375 on, crossing A244, to Shepperton (2 miles).

Shepperton is a pleasant week-end resort on the river, still retaining the nucleus of its old village, round the Church, rebuilt in 1614.

B375 on, crossing the Thames by Chertsey Bridge ($1\frac{1}{2}$ miles), to Chertsey (1 mile).

Chertsey is an agricultural town and a centre of market gardening, with many attractive 17th and 18th century houses in its old-world streets. It was famous for its Benedictine abbey, founded originally in the 7th century. Nothing of this now remains above the ground, though encaustic tiles for which the abbey was well known may be seen in the Parish Church, a building partly of the 14th century, but poorly restored in the 19th century. The charming 18th century Chertsey Bridge is the scene of much riverside activity on fine days in the summer.

A320 (on the left in Chertsey) and B388 (right), skirting St. Anne's Hill, to Thorpe (2 miles), then B389 (left) to Virginia Water ($2\frac{1}{2}$ miles).

Virginia Water, reached by a path behind the Wheatsheaf Hotel, is a beautiful if artificial lake, more than $1\frac{1}{2}$ miles long, surrounded by woods in the southern part of Windsor Great Park (see Tour 2). It was constructed in 1746 by Thomas Sandby, deputy-ranger of the park, for the Duke of Cumberland, later Governor of Virginia. On the south shore is a Roman colonnade from North Africa.

A30 (right), passing the Royal Holloway College, to Egham (on the right; $2\frac{1}{2}$ miles).

Egham is a small country town consisting mainly of one long street, the ends of which are linked by the by-pass road. The Parish Church, rebuilt in 1817 in the classical style, contains 17th-century monuments to the Denhams, and on the galleries are shields placed here by descendants of the barons who stood as sureties for Magna Carta. The massive and elaborate Royal Hollo-

way College for Women, now part of London University, was designed by W. H. Crossland, on the model of a French château, and built in 1879-86.

A308 (left), crossing the field of Runnymede (1 mile), and thence to Old Windsor (3 miles more).

Runnymede, an unfenced meadow $1\frac{1}{2}$ miles long, was the place where Magna Carta, or the Great Charter, designed to combat feudal tyranny, was sealed by King John at the instigation of the barons in 1215. A museum and information centre has been opened by the National Trust here, and a memorial by Sir Edward Maufe, presented by the American Bar Association, commemorates the event. The field is overlooked by the wooded Cooper's Hill, the lovely view from which over the Thames to the Chilterns was extolled by Sir John Denham in a famous poem (1642). On the brow (reached by A328 and a lane on the left) are the Runnymede Air Forces Memorial, designed by Sir Edward Maufe and unveiled in 1953, to the airmen of Britain and the Commonwealth who died in the Second World War and have no known grave, and the National Memorial (by Geoffrey Jellicoe, 1965) to President John F. Kennedy, assassinated in 1963.

A308 on, between Windsor Great Park and the Home Park (on the right), to Windsor ($1\frac{1}{2}$ miles).

Windsor is described in Tour 2 (page 15).

A332 on, crossing the Thames, to Eton ($\frac{1}{2}$ mile).

Eton is a residential town on the north bank of the river, with a narrow winding High Street leading to Eton College, founded in 1440 by Henry VI, the oldest public school in England (after Winchester) and perhaps the most famous. The older buildings, of mellow brick, are arranged round two courts or quadrangles. Over the entrance is Upper School, of the 17th century, with panelling and desks carved with the names of famous Etonians. On the north side of the first court, in Lower School, is the original schoolroom, and on the south is the fine Chapel, built in 1441-61 in the Perpendicular style, with wall paintings of the late 15th century and modern stained glass by Evie Hone and John Piper.

A332 on, under the M4 Motorway, to Slough ($1\frac{1}{2}$ miles).

Slough is a growing residential and industrial town with a large Trading Estate (to the west), established in 1920 and the first of its kind in Britain.

A332 on to Stoke Green ($1\frac{1}{2}$ miles), then B473 (left) and an unclassified road (left again) to the church of Stoke Poges ($\frac{1}{2}$ mile).

Stoke Poges is a scattered residential village. The secluded churchyard is that immortalised in Thomas Gray's Elegy in a Country Churchyard. Outside the east wall of the church is the tomb of his mother, in which the poet himself was buried in 1771. The Church is mainly of the 13th century, with Tudor additions. The unusual manor pew, beneath the tower, is approached from the 16th century Manor House by a private ' cloister '.

B473 on to Farnham Royal (1½ miles), then right to Farnham Common (1½ miles), where roads on the left lead to Burnham Beeches.

Burnham Beeches, a magnificent tract of forest, with many grand old oaks and other trees, was purchased by the Corporation of the City of London in 1880 and added to in 1921-9. The roads in the woodland are many and confusing, and care should be taken to choose a route that returns to B473, which runs on the east side.

B473 on to Beaconsfield (3½ miles).

Beaconsfield, a spreading residential town, retains the nucleus of the old market centre, with wide streets and delightful 18th century houses. In the rebuilt Church, close by, are monuments to Edmund Burke, the statesman, who is buried here.

B473 on northward for 1 mile, then by an unclassified road (right) to Jordans (2 miles more), on the left at a road-junction.

Jordans is famous for its delightfully-secluded Friends' Meeting House, built in 1688. Outside are buried William Penn, the founder of Pennsylvania, his two wives and five of his children, and Thomas Elwood, the friend of Milton. Old Jordans, to the north, a hostel of the Society of Friends, stands on the site of the previous meeting-house, of 1669 or earlier.

Unclassified road north to Butler's Cross (1 mile), then right to Chalfont St. Giles (1 mile).

Chalfont St. Giles is a pleasant residential village in the Misbourne valley, the older part built round a green. The restored 13th-15th century Church here has late-medieval wall paintings. A little above is Milton's Cottage (admission daily, except Tuesdays and Sunday mornings, 10 to 1 and 2.15 to 6 or dusk; in November-January on Saturdays and Sundays only), where John Milton lived in 1665-6 to avoid the Great Plague of London.

Unclassified road on over the river, then A413 (right) to Chalfont St. Peter (2 miles).

Chalfont St. Peter is an expanding residential village, with a few old houses, in the Misbourne valley.

A413 on to Tatling End (3 miles), then A40 (left) for 1 mile; then A412 (left) and an unclassified road (right) to Denham (½ mile).

Denham, on the Misbourne, is a delectable village of 17th and 18th century brick houses, with tiled roofs. Especially notable is Denham Place, at the west end. The restored 15th century Church contains the almost unique brass of an abbess, Agnes Jordan of Syon, who died in 1544.

Unclassified road for ½ mile, then A40 again (left), crossing the Colne valley. A40 on past Northolt Aerodrome and via Greenford and Perivale to Hanger Lane (North Circular Road; 10 miles from Denham), then on via the White City Stadium, Wood Lane (right), Shepherd's Bush, Holland Park Avenue (left) and Bayswater Road to London (Marble Arch; 7 miles).

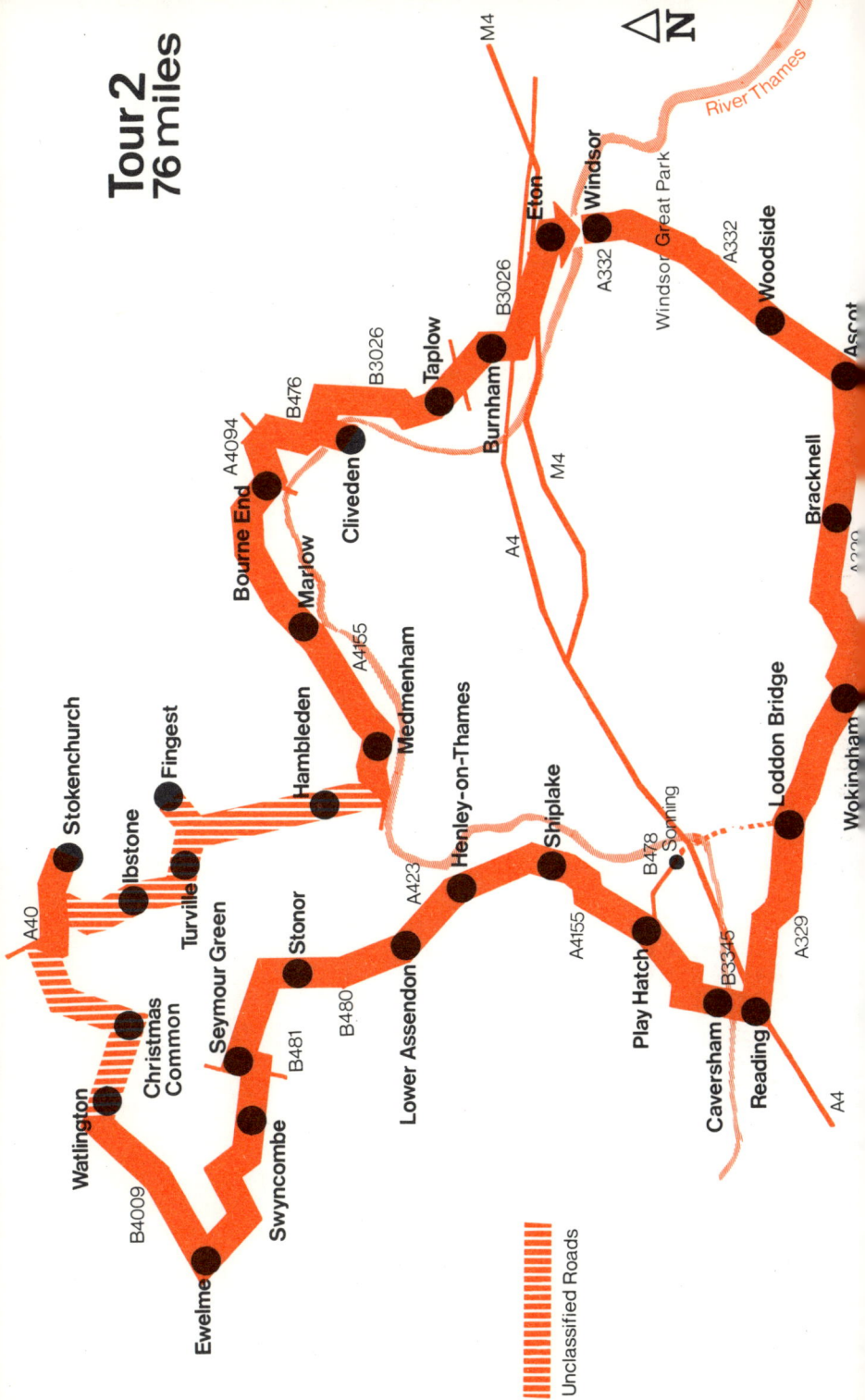

Tour 2
76 miles

N

River Thames

M4

Windsor

Eton

Windsor Great Park

A332

Woodside

Ascot

B3026

Taplow

Burnham

B3026

A332

B476

A4094

Bourne End

Cliveden

M4

Bracknell

A329

Marlow

A4155

A329

Medmenham

Loddon Bridge

Stokenchurch

Fingest

Hambleden

Henley-on-Thames

Shiplake

Wokingham

Ibstone

Turville

Seymour Green

Stonor

A423

Sonning

B478

A40

Christmas Common

B481

B480

Lower Assendon

A4155

Play Hatch

B3345

A329

Watlington

Swyncombe

Caversham

Reading

A4

B4009

Ewelme

Unclassified Roads

2. North-East Berkshire and the Southern Chilterns

This tour starts at Windsor, a historic Thamesside town famous for its royal castle, and crosses the eastern part of Berkshire via Ascot and the new town of Bracknell. It reaches the Thames again at Reading, a busy county and industrial town with a university, then crosses the river and follows it down to Henley, a delightful old town renowned for its royal regatta. From here the tour explores the southern part of the Chiltern Hills, a range of chalk downs, about 36 miles long, extending from the Thames Valley, which separates them from the Berkshire Downs, nearly to Dunstable. The Chilterns show a prominent escarpment towards the north-west, where they face the Vale of Aylesbury, and the southern part is extensively covered by beautiful beech woods. The route takes in the quiet villages of Ewelme (with a notable church), Ibstone, Turville, Fingest and Hambleden, beyond which it reaches the Thames again. It continues through Marlow, another delightful old town, and passes the great house of Cliveden on its way to Eton, famous for its public school, opposite Windsor.

Windsor is an old market town and royal borough, with many fine 17th and 18th century houses, on the south bank of the Thames. From the bridge and the Old House, built for himself by Sir Christopher Wren, Thames Street climbs up round the wall of the castle towards the Guildhall (admission daily, April-October, 1 to 6), completed in 1689 by Wren, with royal portraits and an exhibition of local history. Windsor Castle (admission to precincts daily, 10 to dusk), the principal residence of the sovereign since the 12th century, stands on a chalk cliff rising abruptly from the Thames. It was built originally by William the Conqueror, but has been extended and altered at various times and was extensively restored by Sir Jeffry Wyatville for George IV. Henry VIII's Gateway admits to the Lower Ward or courtyard, in which is St. George's Chapel (admission weekdays 11 to 3.45, Fridays from 1, Sundays 2.30 to 4; closed in January), a magnificent example of the late-Gothic style, with royal tombs, fine glass of about 1500, and a splendid fan-vaulted roof. In the choir are the stalls and banners of the Knights of the Garter, an order instituted in 1348 by Edward III. The adjoining Albert Memorial Chapel, built by Henry VII as his burial-place, was converted by Queen Victoria into a memorial for her consort, Prince Albert, who died in 1861. Above the Lower Ward rises a mound supporting the Round Tower or keep, which commands a wide view, and beyond is the Upper Ward, on the north side of which are the State Apartments (admission in the absence of the court, weekdays 11 to 3, 4 or 5, Sundays in May-October from 1.30). These richly-furnished rooms contain a valuable collection of paintings by Holbein, Rembrandt,

Rubens, Van Dyck and other masters, as well as tapestries, porcelain and many other treasures. In the fine St. George's Hall, remodelled by Wyatville, the ceremonies of the Order of the Garter are held. Near the entrance are Queen Mary's Dolls' House, designed by Sir Edward Lutyens (1923), and an exhibition of Old Master Drawings from the royal collection (admission to both, daily, at the times above).

A332 from High Street, skirting Home Park and crossing Windsor Great Park to Woodside (4½ miles).

Windsor Great Park is a beautiful expanse of well-wooded country extending south from the town, and stocked with fallow deer and a few red deer. Visitors are allowed to wander at will (except in the neighbourhood of the various lodges and where the land is under cultivation), but cars and motor-cycles are prohibited. The park is extended on the north by the private Home Park, which encloses Windsor Castle on its eastward side, and both parks are crossed by the Long Walk, an avenue of chestnuts and planes (planted after the famous elms had to be felled in 1945), leading from the castle to Snow Hill, the highest point in the park, which is surmounted by a huge equestrian statue of George III, familiarly known as " the Copper Horse."

A332 on through Windsor Forest and alongside the racecourse to Ascot (2 miles).

Ascot is a residential town on the heathlands of the Berkshire-Surrey border. Ascot Heath, where horse-racing was started by Queen Anne in 1711, is the scene of the most fashionable meeting of the year (in June), always attended by royalty.

A329 (right) to Bracknell (2½ miles).

Bracknell is an old village that is now absorbed in a New Town, designated in 1949 and intended mainly to attract people and industry away from London. The centre is being rebuilt as a pedestrian precinct and new residential districts are being built from which vehicles are mainly to be excluded. The most successful building architecturally is Point Royal, a 17-storey block of flats designed by Arup Associates (1964), in Rectory Road, to the south-west near the Sandhurst road.

A329 on to Wokingham (4 miles) and thence to Loddon Bridge (3½ miles).

Wokingham is a pleasant residential market town with 17th and 18th century houses in Rose Street and elsewhere. Opposite the Town Hall is the Rose Inn, rebuilt in the 17th century. The restored Parish Church, at the east end, has a 13th century nave with tall chalk piers.

A329 on from Loddon Bridge, crossing A4 and entering Reading (3½ miles) by King's Road and High Street (right).

Reading, the county town of Berkshire, is a thriving and congested commercial and manufacturing place. It has corn and cattle markets and was a centre of the cloth trade from the Middle Ages to the 17th century. To the north of the Market Place is the much-restored 13th-15th century Church of St. Lawrence, which has a tower of 1448, 111 feet high. Adjoining the Town Hall, on its north side, is the Museum and Art Gallery (admission weekdays, 10 to 5.30), with collections of natural history and local history, including architectural details from the abbey and an outstanding display of finds excavated from the large Roman town of Silchester, in Hampshire. Near the Forbury Gardens, east of the church, are the few but imposing remains, including the 14th century gatehouse, of the famous Benedictine Abbey, founded in 1121 by Henry I (who was buried before the high altar). St. Mary's, about ¼ mile west of High Street, is a mainly 16th century church, built in chequered flint and stone, using material from the abbey. In Whiteknights Park, over 1 mile south-east, near the Aldershot road (A327), are the new buildings (from 1947 on) of the University of Reading, founded in 1926. Also in the park is the Museum of English Rural Life (admission Tuesday-Saturday, 10 to 1 and 2 to 4.30), an excellent collection of old vehicles, implements, tools, etc., illustrating agricultural life.

B3345, leaving Reading by The Forbury, across the Thames by Reading Bridge to Caversham (1 mile).

Caversham is a pleasant residential suburb on the north bank of the river, which is a favourite resort for boating.

B3345 on to join A4155 (right) for Play Hatch (2 miles) and thence to Shiplake (2½ miles).

Shiplake, on a high bank above the Thames, has a Victorianised Church in which Lord Tennyson was married in 1850. The 15th century French glass here was brought from the abbey of St. Omer.

A4155 on to Henley-on-Thames (3 miles).

Henley-on-Thames is a delightful town with many fine 18th century brick houses and coaching inns, surrounded by beautiful wooded scenery. The famous Henley Royal Regatta, the chief amateur function of the rowing world, was founded in 1839 and is held in the first week in July. The course of over a mile ends about ¼ mile below the graceful 18th century Bridge. Opposite this is the Red Lion Hotel, on a window of which the poet Shenstone is said to have scratched his celebrated lines, on finding the " warmest welcome at an inn." The large but restored 14th-15th century Church, in Hart Street, the wide main street, has a distinctive 15th century tower. Speaker's House, opposite, is believed to have been the birthplace of William Lenthall, Speaker of the Long Parliament.

A423 north to Lower Assendon (1½ miles), then B480 (right) to Stonor (2½ miles more).

Stonor is a hamlet beautifully situated in a secluded Chiltern valley. Stonor Park (closed at present for restoration), in a deer park on the wooded hill to the east, is a large Tudor and later house. Edmund Campion, the Jesuit martyr, set up his printing press here, and Mass has been said in the chapel close by (visitors usually admitted) for over 800 years.

B480 on, ascending on to the Chiltern plateau, to Seymour Green (3 miles), then B481 (left) to Cookley Green ($\frac{1}{2}$ mile) and by an unclassified road (right) to Swyncombe (1 mile; on the left).

Swyncombe, a hamlet secreted away in a verdant fold of the Chiltern escarpment, has a restored early-Norman Church with an apse.

Unclassified road, below the open Swyncombe Downs, branching right in 2 miles for Ewelme (1 mile).

Ewelme is a charming village in a valley west of the Chiltern Hills. The dignified Church was built after 1430 (embodying a 14th century tower) by William de la Pole, Duke of Suffolk. It contains the splendid tomb of his wife, wearing the Order of the Garter on her left arm. On the floor of the nave and chancel are numerous 15th-17th century brasses, and the 15th century font has a richly-carved cover. In the south chapel, which has a fine timber roof and 15th century stained glass, is the tomb of Thomas Chaucer, believed to be the son of the poet. On the slope below are the excellent brick-built Almshouses and the School, founded by De la Pole in 1437.

B4009 north-east below the Chilterns to Watlington ($3\frac{1}{2}$ miles), then by an unclassified road right, ascending Watlington Hill to Christmas Common ($1\frac{1}{2}$ miles).

Watlington is a small town with a 17th century brick market hall and good 18th century houses. Watlington Hill (750 feet), a spur of the Chiltern escarpment, affords a wide view over the vale of the Thame towards Oxford.

Unclassified road (left) on the wooded Chiltern plateau for $3\frac{1}{2}$ miles, then A40 (right) to Stokenchurch (1 mile).

Stokenchurch is a plain village scattered around several large greens. The Post Office Tower, 320 feet high, on the crest of the ridge to the west, is one of several identical towers in England for television and radio telephony.

Unclassified road south (from the west end of the village) to Ibstone ($2\frac{1}{2}$ miles).

Ibstone is a hamlet in unspoilt Chiltern country, with charming views. The small 12th-13th century Church, on a lane to the right, has a timber belfry and a 15th century pulpit.

Unclassified road on, descending to Turville (over $1\frac{1}{2}$ miles) and thence to Fingest (nearly 1 mile more).

Turville is an attractive hamlet with brick and flint houses in a secluded valley, enclosed by the Chiltern beechwoods. Fingest,

another secluded hamlet, at the head of a long valley, has a 12th-13th century Church with a massive Norman tower capped by an unusual twin saddleback roof (perhaps of the 17th century).

Unclassified road south, down the valley, to Hambleden ($3\frac{1}{2}$ miles).

Hambleden is yet another attractive village, with flint and brick cottages and a 17th century manor house. The long Church, though much restored, is mainly of the 14th century.

Unclassified road on for 1 mile to regain the Thames valley, then A4155 (left) to Medmenham (1 mile).

Medmenham is a residential village on the north bank of the river. At Medmenham Abbey, a large house partly of the 16th century, Sir Francis Dashwood founded the 18th century ' Monks of Medmenham ' (later called the ' Hell-Fire Club '), notorious for the ' blasphemous orgies ' it held.

A4155 on to Marlow (3 miles).

Marlow is a delightful market town, with numerous fine 16th-18th century houses, and a favourite boating resort on the Thames, which is crossed by a charming Suspension Bridge of 1832, restored in 1966. Bourne End (see below) is a large residential village and a popular week-end resort.

A4155 on to Bourne End ($3\frac{1}{2}$ miles), then A4094 (left) for $\frac{1}{2}$ mile, and B476 (right), passing the gates of Cliveden ($1\frac{1}{2}$ miles more).

Cliveden (admission April-October, Wednesdays and Saturdays, 2.30 to 5.30), on a hill whose hanging woods descend steeply to a beautiful reach of the Thames, is a large classical mansion rebuilt in 1851 by Sir Charles Barry, though the interior was altered by J. L. Pearson after its purchase in 1893 by the influential Astor family. It stands on a great terrace which supported the previous house, built for the profligate 2nd Duke of Buckingham, with the delightful gardens below.

B476 on for 2 miles, then B3026 (left) to Taplow ($\frac{1}{2}$ mile) and on across A4 to Burnham Abbey (2 miles more).

Taplow, on the river opposite Maidenhead, has a Church containing the oldest brass of a civilian in England (of about 1350). Burnham Abbey was founded in 1266 for Augustinian canonesses, but the 13th century buildings, rededicated in 1916, are now occupied by a community of Anglican nuns.

B3026 on through Dorney to Eton (3 miles).

Eton is described in Tour 1 (page 12).

A332 across the Thames to Windsor ($\frac{1}{2}$ mile).

Tour 3
103 miles

△ N

Windsor
Eton A332
Slough
Farnham Royal
Farnham Common B473
Beaconsfield
Penn B474
Hazlemere
Princes Risborough A4129
Bledlow A4010
Chinnor B4009
Lambert Arms B4009
Tetsworth A40
Rycote B4013
Great Milton
Cuddesdon B480
Chiselhampton B4015 A423
Dorchester
Shillingford
Benson A423
Crowmarsh Gifford B479
Goring B4009
Mapledurham B4526
Caversham A4155
Sonning A4155
Play Hatch B478 B479
Reading A4
Twyford B3018
Wargrave A321
Hurley A423
Bisham A404
Cookham A4094
Maidenhead A4 B3028
Bray M4
A4
A308
M4 M4

Hughenden
Bradenham
High Wycombe A4128 A40
West Wycombe

River Thames

B4447
A404

Unclassified Roads

3. The Thames above Windsor and the Southern Chilterns

This tour starts (like Tour 2) at the royal borough of Windsor and it explores the Thames Valley upstream as far as Dorchester. It runs through many delightful villages, Bray, Cookham, Hurley, Wargrave, and Sonning, each with its particular points of interest, and beyond the last it crosses the river to Caversham, the northern suburb of Reading. From here it follows the north bank of the Thames, passing near Mapledurham, a secluded village with an Elizabethan house, and Benson, another fine village, to reach Dorchester, yet another charming village, famous for its abbey Church. From here, the route crosses the vale of the Thame (a tributary of the Thames) to reach the Chiltern Hills (see Tour 2). It runs at the foot of the escarpment to Princes Risborough, a pleasant small town, then traverses a beautiful valley of the Chilterns to the delectable villages of Bradenham and West Wycombe and the interesting old town of High Wycombe. A divergence is made to include Hughenden Manor, famous for its association with Disraeli, before returning via Beaconsfield and Eton to Windsor.

Windsor is described in Tour 2 (page 15).

From High Street, via Peascod Street, Oxford Road and A308 to a roundabout serving the M4 Motorway (4½ miles), then B3028 (right) to Bray (½ mile).

Bray is a charming village on the Thames, with the fine brick almshouses of Jesus Hospital, founded in 1627. A 15th century timber-framed church house forms the approach to the restored 14th-15th century Church, which has numerous brasses. The ' Vicar of Bray ' of the famous ballad was Francis Carswell, who held his post from Charles II to Queen Anne, though the legend was first attached to Simon Aleyn, who " thrice changed his creed to keep his preferment " under the last four Tudor monarchs.

B3028 on to Maidenhead (1½ miles).

Maidenhead is a residential town and a favoured boating resort on a beautiful reach of the river, here crossed by a graceful 18th century bridge. Boulter's Lock, upstream, is especially popular at summer week-ends. Oldfield, a house in Riverside, south of the bridge, now contains the Henry Reitlinger Bequest (admission Tuesdays and Thursdays, 10 to 12.30 and 2.15 to 4.30), an art collection notable for its Oriental ceramics and drawings. The town centre, with St. Mary's Church (rebuilt in 1965 by Lord Mottistone), is ¾ mile west of the bridge, on A4.

A4 (right) to Maidenhead Bridge (see above), then A4094 (left), passing Boulter's Lock, to Cookham (2½ miles).

Cookham, facing the Cliveden woods (Tour 2), beyond the Thames, is a village with attractive cottages and inns, and a popular week-end resort. Sir Stanley Spencer was born (in 1891) and spent most

21

of his life at Cookham; the Stanley Spencer Gallery contains a selection of paintings and drawings, and in the medieval Church is a Last Supper by him.

B4447 (left) for $\frac{1}{2}$ mile, then by an unclassified road (right) over Winter Hill, descending by zigzags to the river south of Marlow Bridge ($3\frac{1}{2}$ miles; Tour 2), then A404 (left) to Bisham ($\frac{1}{2}$ mile).

Bisham has a Victorianised Church notable for its 16th and 17th century monuments of the Hoby family. Bisham Abbey, on the river bank, upstream, is a mainly Tudor mansion that is now a centre of the Central Council of Physical Recreation.

A404 on for $1\frac{1}{2}$ miles, then A423 (right) for Hurley (1 mile; on the right).

Hurley is an attractive village on the Thames, with a timbered 15th century inn and a restored Church which shows Saxon and Norman work. This became part of a Benedictine priory of which other remains are the refectory, incorporated in a house on the north side, and two large stone barns and a circular dovecote.

A423 on for $1\frac{1}{2}$ miles, then by an unclassified road left via Holly Cross to Wargrave (3 miles).

Wargrave is a delightful village much favoured by artists. The Church near the river, burned down by Suffragettes, was rebuilt in 1916, when Norman masonry was discovered beneath the 17th century brickwork of the tower.

A321 south, crossing A4, to Twyford (2 miles).

Twyford is a large village with several 18th century houses. The church of Ruscombe, $\frac{3}{4}$ mile east, has a Norman chancel (with 13th century wall paintings) and a tower and nave of 1639.

B3018 (right) from Twyford to reach A4 (1 mile), then B478 on to Sonning (1 mile more).

Sonning is another delightful village, with an attractive old bridge and lock, and a variety of flower-decorated houses. The 13th-14th century Church, though much Victorianised, has numerous brasses.

B478 on over the Thames to Play Hatch ($1\frac{1}{2}$ miles) and A4155 (left) thence to Caversham ($1\frac{1}{2}$ miles; on Tour 2), then B479 on for $2\frac{1}{2}$ miles and B 4526 (left) to Trench Green ($\frac{1}{2}$ mile), from which a narrow lane descends to Mapledurham (over 1 mile farther).

Mapledurham, a hamlet in charming seclusion on the Thames, has a weir and water-mill popular with artists. The Church has a Norman font and a clock given by William III. The south aisle is walled off as the Roman Catholic chapel of Mapledurham House (admission Easter-September, Saturdays, Sundays and Bank Holiday Mondays and Tuesdays, 2.30 to 5.30), a well-restored Elizabethan manor house, built in 1568, long the home of the Blount family that included Martha Blount, the friend of Alexander Pope. Their portraits (probably by Kneller) are among the paintings.

B4526 on from Trench Green, among pleasant woodlands, to Goring (6 miles).

Goring is a large village on the Thames, at the entrance to the gap which it makes between the Chiltern Hills and the Berkshire Downs. The partly Norman Church, on the road to the bridge to Streatley (on Tour 4), has a vaulted Norman tower with a rare tourelle, or round stair turret.

B4009 north via South Stoke to the entrance to Carmel College ($4\frac{1}{2}$ miles), then B479 on to Crowmarsh Gifford (1 mile).

Crowmarsh Gifford, on the Thames opposite Wallingford (Tour 4), has a complete, if restored, Norman Church. Carmel College is a Jewish public school with a striking synagogue designed in 1964 by Tom Hancock. Howbery Park, where Jethro Tull, the 18th century pioneer of mechanised agriculture, lived, is now the Hydraulics Research Station of the Ministry of Technology.

A4130 (left) and A423 (right), passing Howbery Park, to Benson (2 miles; on the right).

Benson, once the seat of the Kings of Mercia, is an attractive village with several old inns, near a large R.A.F. Station.

A423 on to Shillingford (1 mile) and thence to Dorchester ($1\frac{1}{2}$ miles more).

Dorchester, a village on the Thame near its junction with the Thames, has a pleasing variety of old houses and inns. It was an important Saxon town, the cathedral centre of Wessex from 634 to 705, when the bishopric was moved to Winchester, then of Mercia from 869 to 1072, when the see was transferred to Lincoln. The interesting Abbey Church is actually that of a priory of Augustinian Canons founded in 1140. It is mainly in the Transitional Norman style of the late 12th century and the Decorated style of the late 13th and 14th centuries. The choir aisles open from beautiful arcades and the east end of the choir has three remarkable windows, the unusual tracery of which is sculptured with figures and contains 14th century stained glass. The east window was restored in 1966 as a memorial to Sir Winston Churchill. Under the south window are fine canopied sedilia and piscina; the early (12th century) glass in the small windows here shows scenes from the life of St. Birinus, the founder of the first Saxon cathedral. The church has 14th century monuments and a Norman lead font with eleven figures of the Apostles. The timber south porch is a 15th century addition and the west tower is of the 17th century.

A423 on for $2\frac{1}{2}$ miles, then B4015 (right) to Chiselhampton ($2\frac{1}{2}$ miles).

Chiselhampton, a hamlet on the Thame, has a handsome Manor House of 1768 and an unspoilt Georgian Church of 1763 with its original furnishings.

B480 (left) for 1 mile, then by an unclassified road (right) via Denton to Cuddesdon (2 miles more).

Cuddesdon, well situated on a hill above the Thame, has a 12th-15th century Church, a Theological College founded in 1854 by Bishop Samuel Wilberforce, and the Palace of the Bishop of Oxford, rebuilt in a modest style in 1962.

Unclassified road (right), crossing the Thame, then branching right and left to Great Milton (2 miles).

Great Milton has fine stone houses and thatched cottages, and a restored 13th-15th century Church with good 14th century window tracery and a splendid 17th century monument.

Unclassified road south from the church, then B4013 (left) to the Three Pigeons Inn (2 miles; from which the road goes on to the entrance to Rycote, 1 mile farther); then A40 (right) through Tetsworth to the Lambert Arms Hotel (5½ miles).

Rycote consists of a house rebuilt in 1911, out of the stables of its 16th century forerunner, and a well-restored 15th century Chapel (admission 9.30 to 4, 5.30 or 7, Sundays from 2), which has interesting 15th and 17th century woodwork, including two elaborately-carved family pews.

B4009 (left) from the Lambert Arms, at the foot of the finely wooded Chiltern Hills, to Chinnor (2½ miles) and thence to Bledlow (2 miles; to the right).

Chinnor has large cement works and a good 14th century Church with numerous brasses and sixteen paintings of saints by Sir James Thornhill. Bledlow has paper mills and brick houses, and a church, mostly of the 13th-14th centuries, with a richly-sculptured Norman font of the Aylesbury type.

B4009 on for 2 miles, then A4129 (right) to Princes Risborough (1 mile).

Princes Risborough is a small town below the Chilterns, with old buildings, including the tiny Town Hall of 1824 and the fine 17th century Manor House (admission Tuesdays and Wednesdays, 2.30 to 4.30). The much-restored Church has some good 13th century work. Whiteleaf Cross, cut in the chalk escarpment to the east, is 80 feet long but of unknown age.

A4010 south through a lovely Chiltern valley to Bradenham (4½ miles).

Bradenham is pleasingly scattered round a large green. The Church, though mostly of the 15th century, has a Saxon or early Norman doorway. The large brick 17th century Manor House was the home of Isaac D'Israeli, the father of Lord Beaconsfield (see below).

A4010 on to West Wycombe (1½ miles; to the right on A40).

West Wycombe (now happily by-passed) is perhaps the most enchanting of all the Chiltern villages, with 15th-18th century houses, mostly of brick and timber. To the south, in charmingly

landscaped grounds, is West Wycombe Park (admission July and August, Tuesday-Sunday and Bank Holiday Monday, 2.15 to 6), a house remodelled in about 1735-70 by Sir Francis Dashwood, founder of the ' Hell-Fire Club ' (see Medmenham), who was visited here in 1773 by Benjamin Franklin, the American author. In the side of the chalk hill north of the village are the artificial ' Hell-Fire ' Caves, where the club is supposed to have held its ' orgies ' and on the summit is the Church, practically rebuilt by Dashwood, with unusual furnishings and a tower surmounted by a gilded ball (a prominent landmark from the High Wycombe road) capable of holding about ten persons.

A40 (left) through the Wye valley to High Wycombe (2 miles).

High Wycombe is a prosperous market and industrial town famous for its manufacture of chairs and other furniture (originally from the Chiltern beechwoods). The delightful Guildhall, closing the west end of High Street, was built in 1757; from the porch of the Red Lion Inn, close by, Benjamin Disraeli made his first political speech. The 13th and 15th century Parish Church, north of the Cornmarket, has a tower completed in the 18th century and a spacious interior with notable monuments. The Art Gallery and Museum (admission weekdays, except Wednesday, 10 to 5.30, 6 or 8), in Castle Hill, has a good collection of decorative woodwork.

A4128 north from Church Street, skirting the park of Hughenden Manor ($1\frac{1}{2}$ miles).

Hughenden Manor (admission Tuesday-Friday and Bank Holiday Mondays, 2 to 6; Saturdays and Sundays 10 to 1 and 2 to 6; closed Bank Holiday Tuesdays and in January), on the side of a wooded valley, is a late 18th century house remodelled for Benjamin Disraeli, Earl of Beaconsfield, whose home it was from 1848 until his death in 1881. It was reopened in 1949 as a memorial museum, and has numerous portraits and relics. In the Church below is a memorial to Lord Beaconsfield, presented by Queen Victoria, and the statesman is buried in the churchyard.

A4128 on to Cryers Hill (1 mile), then by an unclassified road (right) via Widmer End to Hazlemere (2 miles), on A404, then B474 to Penn ($2\frac{1}{2}$ miles).

Penn, perhaps the ancestral home of William Penn, the coloniser, is a high-lying village on the Chilterns, with a partly-medieval Church that has a rare lead font and an unusual 15th century ' Doom ' painted on boards.

B474 on to Beaconsfield (3 miles) and B473 on again, beyond A40, to Farnham Common (for Burnham Beeches; $3\frac{1}{2}$ miles) and thence via Farnham Royal to the Slough Trading Estate (3 miles); then A4 (left) to Slough (1 mile) and A332 (right) to Eton ($1\frac{1}{2}$ miles) and thence to Windsor ($\frac{1}{2}$ mile).

Beaconsfield, Burnham Beeches, Slough and Eton are all described in Tour 1 (pages 12-13).

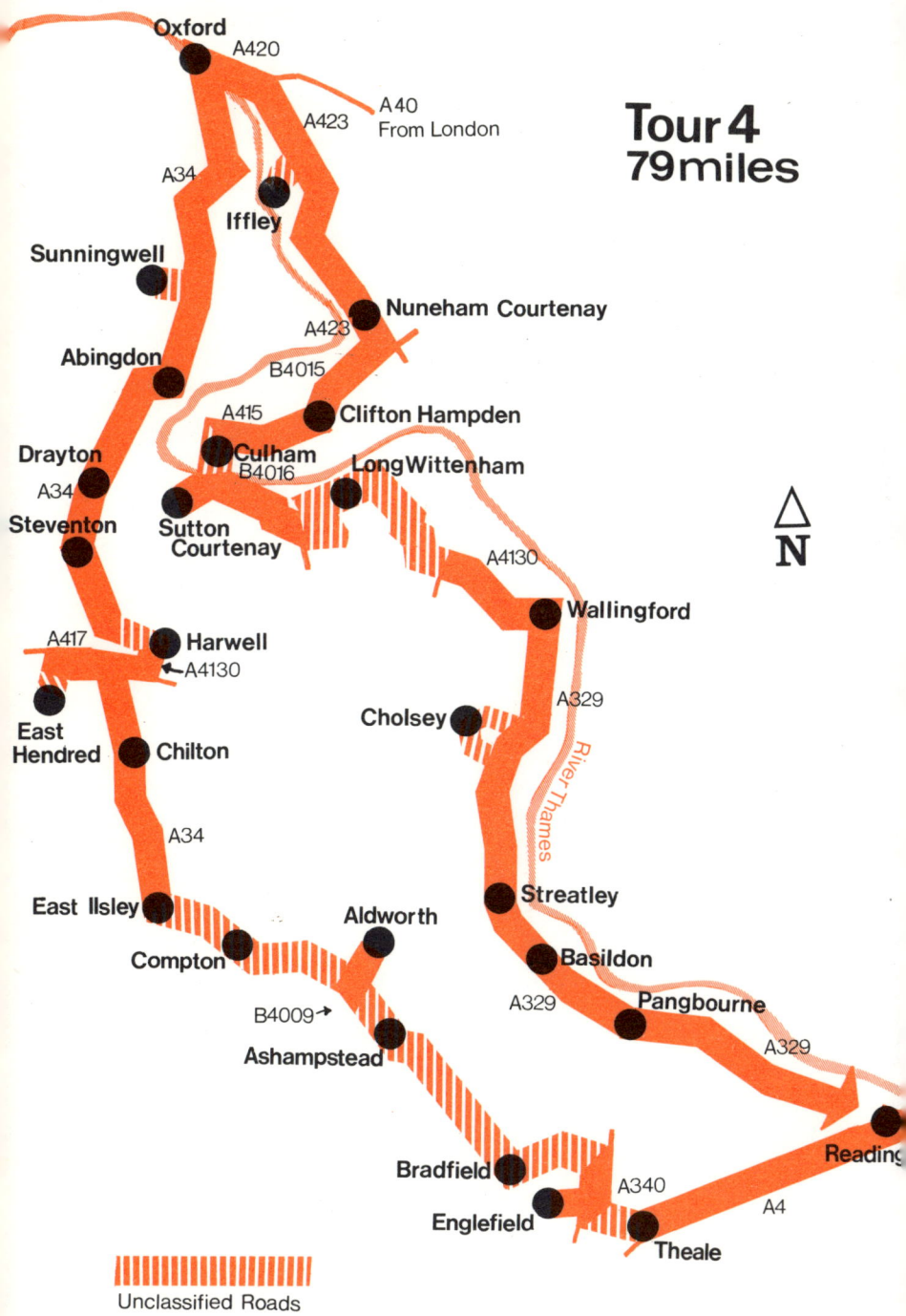

Oxford

A420

A40
From London

A423

Tour 4
79 miles

A34

Iffley

Sunningwell

Nuneham Courtenay

A423

Abingdon

B4015

Clifton Hampden

A415

Culham

Long Wittenham

Drayton

B4016

A34

Sutton
Courtenay

Steventon

A4130

Wallingford

A417

Harwell

A4130

A329

East
Hendred

Chilton

Cholsey

River Thames

A34

Streatley

East Ilsley

Aldworth

Basildon

Compton

A329

Pangbourne

B4009

A329

Ashampstead

Reading

Bradfield

A340

Englefield

A4

Theale

N

Unclassified Roads

4. The Berkshire Downs and the Thames below Oxford

This tour, starting from the thriving county and industrial town of Reading, ascends the Kennet valley at first, then crosses the eastern reaches of the Berkshire Downs, the long range of chalk downs that extends the Chiltern Hills west of the Thames gap. From East Ilsley it drops down the escarpment which faces over the Vale of White Horse. The route goes through the delightful villages of East Hendred, Harwell, and Steventon and the charming old town of Abingdon, on the Thames, before reaching Oxford. The tour descends the Thames valley via Iffley, with its excellent Norman church, crosses the river to Sutton Courtenay, another delightful village, then goes on to Wallingford, an important Thamesside town in Saxon times, from which it follows the south bank via Streatley and Pangbourne back to Reading.

Reading is described in Tour 2 (page 17).

A4, leaving Reading on the south-west via Minster Street, Castle Street and Bath Road, through the Kennet valley to Theale (5 miles), then by an unclassified road (right) and A340 (right again) to Englefield (1 mile; on the left).

Englefield is a small village consisting of a single street of model cottages leading to the fine deer park of Englefield House, an Elizabethan mansion partly rebuilt after a fire in 1886.

A340 on for $\frac{1}{2}$ mile, then by an unclassified road (left) to Bradfield (2 miles more).

Bradfield is on the small river Pang. Adjoining the village are the brick and flint buildings of Bradfield College, a public school founded in 1850.

Unclassified road (right), crossing the river, then branching left in 1 mile and ascending through pleasant woodlands to Ashampstead (4 miles; to the left); then on to join B4009 for Aldworth ($1\frac{1}{2}$ miles).

Ashampstead has a 13th century Church with contemporary wall paintings. At Aldworth the 14th century church is remarkable for its series of mutilated effigies of the De La Beche family, all under canopies that have been elaborately restored.

B4009 back and by an unclassified road (right; the continuation of the Bradfield road), over a more open section of the Berkshire Downs to Compton ($2\frac{1}{2}$ miles), and thence to East Ilsley (2 miles).

Compton has the field station of the Agricultural Research Council. East Ilsley, in a valley of the downs, was once an important sheep market and is now noted for the training of racehorses.

A34 (right), climbing to Gore Hill, on the ridge of the downs, then down to Chilton (3 miles). A34 on to the crossing of A417 (2 miles), then left on that road for East Hendred (2 miles), on an unclassified road to the left.

East Hendred is a charming village with many old houses and a rare 15th century wayside Chapel with a priest's house attached to it. The Church, though over-restored, has a good 15th century tower, 13th century nave arcades with carved capitals, and a unique 14th century wooden lectern of two tiers. Hendred House, close by, is partly medieval, and incorporates a chapel where Mass has been celebrated since the 13th century.

A417 back, crossing A34, then A4130 (left) to Harwell ($2\frac{1}{2}$ miles).

Harwell, which gives its name to the Atomic Energy Establishment, is a pleasant village among cherry and other orchards. Milton (see below) has a fine 17th-18th century Manor House (open May to September, Saturdays, Sundays and Bank Holidays, 2.30 to 6) with an 18th century Gothic library and chapel, in a wooded park.

Unclassified road left from Harwell, then A34 (right) to Milton Hill ($1\frac{1}{2}$ miles; from which Milton is $1\frac{1}{2}$ miles right by an unclassified road) and thence to Steventon ($2\frac{1}{2}$ miles).

Steventon has many delightful timber-framed houses and a green crossed by an unusual raised and paved causeway. Priory Cottages (admission Wednesdays, 2 to 6), at the west end of the long street, incorporate the great hall of a Benedictine priory.

A34 on to Drayton ($1\frac{1}{2}$ miles).

Drayton, in the flat meadowlands that open from the Thames to the Vale of White Horse, is an attractive village whose Church contains carvings from a 15th century alabaster reredos.

A34 on to Abingdon ($2\frac{1}{2}$ miles).

Abingdon is an interesting old agricultural town on the Thames which developed under the dominance of a wealthy Benedictine abbey and was later an important centre of the wool trade. In the Market Place is the splendid County Hall, built in 1678-82 by Christopher Kempster, Wren's master-mason on St. Paul's Cathedral. The spacious upper chamber, used as the sessions hall for Berkshire until 1869 (when Reading became the county town), now contains a small museum of local history (admission daily, 2.30 to 6). Facing it is the 13th-15th century Church of St. Nicholas, and to the south of this is the Guildhall, mostly of the 18th century, but embodying part of the abbey hospital and the old Grammar School, founded in 1563. The 15th century Abbey Gatehouse, close by, gives access to the other surviving buildings of the abbey (admission weekdays, 11 to 1 and 2 to 6 or dusk; Sundays, 2.30 to 5.30), including the 13th century Checker, or Exchequer, with a rare contemporary chimney, the 14th century Checker Hall (now fitted up as a theatre), and the 15th-16th century Long Gallery, which is open on one side. East St. Helen Street, with many fine 18th century and older houses, leads from the Market Place to St. Helen's, a 15th century Church with double aisles, making it

wider than it is long. It has a 13th century porch-tower with a 15th century spire, 150 feet high, and on the roof of the north chapel is a unique series of 14th century figure paintings. The churchyard is enclosed by 15th-18th century ranges of almshouses.

A34 on, crossing the ring road and the Thames to Oxford ($6\frac{1}{2}$ miles), which is entered by St. Aldate's.

Oxford is described in Tour 5 (pages 31-33).

A420, extending the High Street east over Magdalen Bridge, then A423 (right) for $1\frac{1}{2}$ miles and by an unclassified road (right again) to Iffley ($\frac{1}{2}$ mile).

Iffley, now a residential suburb of Oxford, has perhaps the finest late Norman parish church in England, an aisleless building with a square central tower, supported by elaborate arches with unusual zigzag moulding, and a west front with a richly-ornamented doorway. The massive black marble font is also Norman, but the rounded apse has been replaced by a 13th century square end.

Unclassified road back, then right on A423 to Nuneham Courtenay (4 miles).

Nuneham Courteney village was moved to a new position on the main road in 1765 by the Earls of Harcourt, whose estate, Nuneham Park, with fine woods bordering the Thames, now belongs to Oxford University.

A423 for 1 mile, then B4015 (right) to Clifton Hampden ($1\frac{1}{2}$ miles).

Clifton Hampden is an attractive village whose restored 12th-14th century Church is charmingly placed on a bank above the river.

A415 (right) to Culham ($2\frac{1}{2}$ miles; on the left).

Culham is likewise on the Thames. Before reaching it, the main road passes the Culham Laboratory of the Atomic Energy Authority and Culham College, a training college of the Church of England, founded in 1853.

Unclassified road across the Thames to Sutton Courtenay (1 mile), to the right on B4016.

Sutton Courtenay is a charming village with 16th-18th century houses, on a backwater of the Thames. On the edge of the green is the 12th-15th century Church, which has a 16th century brick porch, and nearly opposite is Norman Hall, a manor house partly of about 1200. The 15th century and later Manor House, to the south-west, and the Abbey, embodying remains of a 14th century Benedictine grange, are now a home of the Ockenden Venture for helping displaced persons from abroad.

B4016 back (east) through Appleford for $3\frac{1}{2}$ miles, then by an unclassified road (left) to Long Wittenham (1 mile).

Long Wittenham, on another backwater, is an attractive village with thatched and timbered cottages. At the west end of the long street is the Pendon Museum (admission Saturdays, Sundays and Bank Holidays, 3 to 6.15) of Miniature Landscape and Transport, recreating the rural life of about 1930 in models. The 12th-14th century Church, near the east end, has a late-Norman lead font and a remarkable 13th century piscina combined with the tiny effigy of a knight. Beyond Little Wittenham (see below) the road traverses the twin Sinodun Hills, crowned by the Wittenham Clumps of beeches, a prominent landmark in the Thames valley.

Unclassified road (right) beyond Long Wittenham Church, via Little Wittenham (1½ miles), then left to join A4130 (in 1½ miles), which goes on to Wallingford (2 miles more).

Wallingford, a market town and riverside resort, was one of the most important towns in England in Saxon and Norman times, and is still partly enclosed (on the west) by earthen ramparts, probably of Saxon origin. In the Market Place is the picturesque 17th century Town Hall, and south of this is St. Mary's, one of the three survivors of the fourteen medieval churches. High Street, to the north, with the 16th century timber-framed George Hotel, leads to the long Bridge of sixteen arches which crosses the Thames to Crowmarsh Gifford (on Tour 3). To the north of the street, in private grounds, are the few remains of the Norman Castle, where Henry II (who incorporated the town in 1155) held his first parliament. In Thames Street, which has good 18th century houses, are St. Peter's, a church rebuilt in 1769-77, and St. Leonard's, which has fine Norman arches and much pseudo-Norman restoration.

A329 south, following the river, to Cholsey (2 miles; on the right).

Cholsey is a large residential village. The fine cruciform Church, over a mile from the main road, on the South Moreton road, is basically Norman, but has a 13th century chancel extension.

A329 on via Moulsford to Streatley (4 miles).

Streatley is an attractive village opposite Goring (on Tour 3), at the point where the Thames enters the distinctive gap between the charmingly wooded Berkshire Downs and the Chiltern Hills.

A329 on to Basildon (1½ miles).

Basildon is on a beautiful reach of the Thames. The ornamental gardens (admission daily in summer) of the Child-Beale Trust (on a lane to the left) have ornamental pavilions, sculpture and aviaries.

A329 on to Pangbourne (2½ miles).

Pangbourne is another attractive village (though becoming suburbanised) and a boating resort on the Thames. The Gothic Church of 1866 retains a brick tower of 1718.

A329 on to Reading (6 miles), which is entered by Oxford Road and Broad Street.

5. Oxford, the Eastern Cotswolds and the Cherwell Valley

Starting from the historic university of Oxford, this tour follows A34, the Stratford road, passing near Bladon churchyard, the burial-place of Sir Winston Churchill, and Blenheim Palace, the grandiose mansion built for the Duke of Marlborough, ancestor of Sir Winston, who was born here. Beyond the charming small town of Woodstock and the entrance to Ditchley Park, it turns off to explore a quiet and little-known section of the Cotswold country, taking in the lovely ironstone village of Great Tew, Bloxham with its beautiful Church, and the medieval and Elizabethan Broughton Castle. From the fine old market town of Banbury, the route goes on to Sulgrave, famous for its associations with the ancestors of President Washington. The return to Oxford is made by way of Brackley, another fine town, and the delightful villages of King's Sutton, Adderbury and Deddington, and then down the valley of the Cherwell, passing the 17th century Rousham House.

Oxford, famous for its historic university, is one of the most interesting and fascinating cities in England. The " city of dreaming spires " is renowned chiefly for the Gothic architecture of its colleges, with their picturesque halls, chapels and libraries, their sequestered ' quads ' and quiet gardens, but it has also many non-collegiate buildings of great interest. Lying in an open valley on the upper Thames, just above the point where it is joined by the Cherwell (or ' Char '), Oxford is also a county borough and the seat of a bishop, and has thriving motor works established in 1912 by William Morris, the late Lord Nuffield. Oxford University has 35 colleges, of which five are for women only; the halls, chapels and quadrangles of most of them are usually open to visitors (especially between about 10 and 5). University College, one of the three that claim to be the oldest at Oxford, was first endowed in 1249, though statutes granting self-government were not issued until 1280. Balliol College was founded about 1260, but in this case the first statutes were not granted until 1282. Merton College was founded in 1264 and it retains many of the 13th century buildings, notably the chapel with its painted glass, and the 14th century library is the most interesting medieval library in the country. St. Edmund Hall, also founded in the 13th century, is the sole survivor of the medieval halls, forerunners of the colleges, but it has enjoyed full collegiate status since 1937. Christ Church, the largest College in Oxford, was endowed in 1525 by Cardinal Wolsey and refounded by Henry VIII in 1546, when the chapel became the seat of the new bishopric of Oxford (see below). St Catherine's College, founded in 1868 as the St. Catherine's Society to look after the interests of non-collegiate students, occupies a fine building by Arne Jacobsen (1964). Among the many non-collegiate buildings of interest in Oxford, one of the most important is the Bodleian

From Stratford-upon-Avon
and Birmingham

Sulgrave

B4525

A422

Helmdon

A422

Middleton Cheney

B4035

Banbury

From
Northampton

A43

Broughton
Castle

King's
Sutton

A41

Brackley

Bloxham

A43

A361

Adderbury

South
Newington

A423

Deddington

Great Tew

A43

B4022

Steeple Aston

N

B4030

B4030

Enstone

Rousham
House

Middleton Stoney

A34

Ditchley Park

A43

Weston-on-the-Green

Woodstock

A34

A43

Blenheim Palace

Kidlington

Bladon

A4095

Yarnton

A423

B4449

A34

Tour 5
83 miles

Oxford

A40

From London

Unclassified Roads

University Museum

St. John's College (1555)

Wadham College (1612)

MANSFIELD RD.

A43 A24

ST. GILES

PARKS ROAD

Ashmolean Museum

Trinity College (1554)

St. Catherine's College (1868)

CROSS ROAD

Worcester College (1714)

BEAUMONT ST.

HOLYWELL STREET

Balliol College (1260)

Hertford College (1740)

New College (1379)

GEORGE STREET

BROAD ST.

All Souls College (1438)

The Queen's College (1340)

Magdalen College (1458)

LONG WALL

CORNMARKET ST.

TURL STREET

Bodleian Library

A420 To London

Jesus College (1571)

NEW ROAD

Nuffield College (1937)

A420

QUEEN ST.

ST. ALDATES

HIGH STREET

University College (1249)

Oriel College (1326)

MERTON STREET

Merton College (1264)

Christ Church (1525)

Pembroke College (1624)

Cathedral

OXFORD

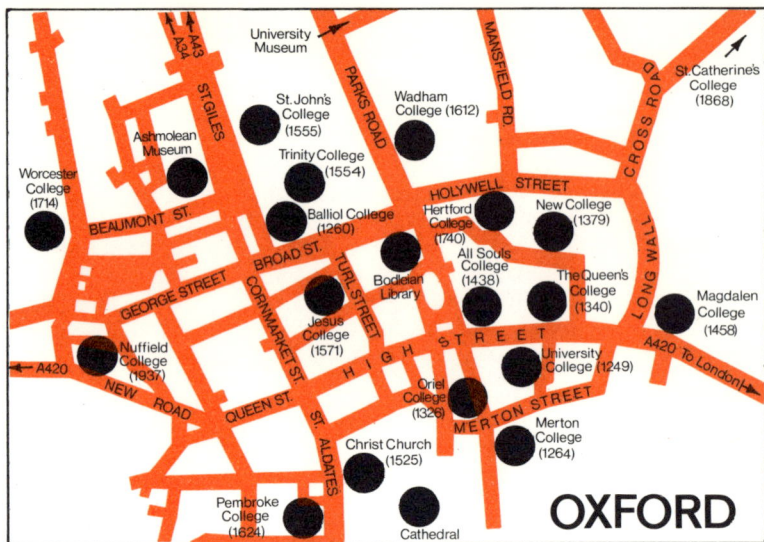

Library, second only to that of the British Museum. Founded in 1602 by Sir Thomas Bodley, it has a large extension with an Exhibition Room (admission Monday-Friday 10 to 1 and 2 to 5; Saturdays 10 to 12.30), opened in 1946. The distinctive Radcliffe Camera, a classical rotunda by James Gibbs, completed in 1749 as a library, is now part of the Bodleian. The Divinity School close by is a superb example of 15th century building notable for its vaulted stone ceiling. The Sheldonian Theatre (admission weekdays, 10 to 12.45 and 2 to 4 or 5, including the Divinity School), designed by Wren (1669), and the Clarendon Building, by Nicholas Hawksmoor (1713), are both now used for various university functions. The Ashmolean Museum (admission usually weekdays 10 to 4, Sundays 2 to 4), an outstanding museum of art and archaeology and the oldest public collection in England (1683), contains many priceless treasures. The Old Ashmolean Museum (admission weekdays, 10.30 to 1 and 2.30 to 4), its original home, now houses the interesting Museum of the History of Science. The University Museum (admission weekdays, 10 to 4), opened in 1860, contains the natural science collections; and the Pitt Rivers Museum (admission weekdays, 2 to 4) is an important museum of ethnology. The Cathedral (admission daily, 11 to 5), originally the chapel of Christ Church (see above), is a fine example of Norman architecture, though the west end was altered by Wolsey. It has a beautiful 15th century stone-vaulted ceiling in the choir. A late-Norman doorway in the Cloisters admits to the lovely 13th century Chapter House, now used for divinity lectures. The 13th century spire of the cathedral is said to be the earliest in England. Notable among the other churches of Oxford are St. Michael's, which has an early-Norman tower; St. Peter's-in-the-East, remarkable for its Norman

crypt; and (best of all) St. Mary the Virgin, the university church since the 14th century at least. Mainly of 15th century construction, it has an ornate 14th century spire and an unusual 17th century baroque porch. On the north-east is the Old Congregation House, which housed the first university library (1320). At the east end of the High Street, perhaps the most beautiful street in England, and close to the fine 18th century Magdalen Bridge is the Botanic Garden (admission weekdays 7.30 to 5, Sundays 10 to 12 and 2 to 4.30 or 6), the oldest of its kind in the country (1621).

A34, leaving Oxford (Carfax) via Magdalen Street, St. Giles', and Woodstock Road, and crossing the by-pass to A4095 (7 miles), which leads left for nearly 1 mile to Bladon.

Bladon Churchyard has become a goal of pilgrimage since Sir Winston Churchill (see below) was buried here, among his ancestors, in 1965.

A34 on, passing an entrance to Blenheim Palace ($\frac{1}{2}$ mile).

Blenheim Palace (admission April-October, Monday-Thursday, 1 to 6; also Easter week-end and Saturdays and Sundays from late July to mid-September; closed during Spring Bank Holiday week-end), the vast and ponderous masterpiece of Sir John Vanbrugh, was begun in 1705 for John Churchill, 1st Duke of Marlborough, as a royal reward for his victory over the French and Bavarians at Blenheim, and was completed after the duke's death, in 1722. The State Rooms are remarkable for their wall and ceiling paintings, their tapestries of the duke's victories, and the family portraits by Kneller, Reynolds and others, and in the Chapel is the ornate marble monument of the duke and his redoubtable duchess (Sarah Jennings). Sir Winston Churchill, a direct descendant of the duke, was born in one of the smaller rooms, in 1874. The large deer park includes some noble oaks and a lake constructed by ' Capability ' Brown.

A34 on to Woodstock ($\frac{1}{2}$ mile).

Woodstock is a delightful small town, noted for its glove-making, near an approach to the palace. It has a Town Hall of 1766 and a Church with an 18th century tower, and in the streets are many houses and shop fronts of about the same period. Fletcher's House, partly Elizabethan, was opened in 1966 as the Oxford City and County Museum (admission weekdays 10 to 5 or 6, Sundays in May-September, 2 to 6), illustrating the geology, industry, agriculture and domestic life of the county.

A34 on, passing the entrance to Ditchley Park (4 miles), over 1 mile to the left, and thence to Enstone (3 miles).

Ditchley Park (admission daily, 2 to 5, for about a fortnight in late July and early August), a fine 18th century classical house by James Gibbs, is notable for its interior decoration by William Kent and Henry Flitcroft. During the Second World War, it was the week-end headquarters of Sir Winston Churchill, and it is now

34

an Anglo-American conference centre. Enstone is a pleasant limestone village in the Glyme valley, with a church showing work of every period from the 12th to the 15th century.

B4030 (right), passing the church, then B4022 (left) to Great Tew (3½ miles), on the right.

Great Tew is a delectable village of ironstone cottages, thatched and stone-roofed, in a setting of fine old trees.

B4022 on for 1 mile, then A361 (right) to South Newington (2 miles more).

South Newington, pleasantly situated in the Swere valley, has a Church, partly of the 12th and 13th centuries, with extensive series of 14th century wall paintings.

A361 on to Bloxham (2 miles).

Bloxham is an attractive village containing the buildings of Bloxham School, a public school founded in 1860. The splendid Church, mostly of the 13th and 14th centuries, has a finely decorated late 14th century spire, a spacious chapel with large windows added in the 15th century and a 15th century rood-screen with painted panels.

A361 on to Banbury (3½ miles).

Banbury, in the valley of the Cherwell is a thriving market and industrial town, famous for its cakes and ale. The Parish Church was rebuilt in 1797-1822 by S. P. Cockerell in a classical style. At the south end of the Horse Fair is the Banbury Cross of the nursery rhyme, rebuilt in 1859 (the original was destroyed by Puritans in 1602).

A422 on from the cross to Middleton Cheney (3½ miles), to the left.

Middleton Cheney is an ironstone village whose restored Church has a fine 15th century tower and spire, and windows filled with glowing stained glass by William Morris to designs by himself, Burne-Jones, F. M. Brown and others.

Unclassified road, passing the church, for ½ mile, then B4525 (right) via Thorpe Mandeville for 3½ miles more, then by an unclassified road (right again) to Sulgrave (½ mile).

Sulgrave is described in Tour 7 (page 45).

Unclassified road south-east from the church to Helmdon (3 miles), then south to join A43 in 3½ miles, about 1 mile short of Brackley.

Brackley is described in Tour 6 (page 40).

A43 on for 1 mile, then by an unclassified road (right) via Charlton to Kings' Sutton (5 miles).

King's Sutton is a pleasant ironstone village in the open Cherwell valley. The Church, mainly of the 12th-14th centuries, has a 15th century west porch, a splendid 14th century tower with unusual pinnacles and a 15th century spire, 198 feet high.

Unclassified road, crossing the river, for $2\frac{1}{2}$ miles, then A41 (left) and A423 on to Adderbury ($\frac{1}{2}$ mile).

Adderbury is a charming village with many fine ironstone houses, including the 17th century Adderbury House, the home of the poet Earl of Rochester, which is passed on the way to the Church, a noble cruciform building, mostly of the 13th and 14th centuries, with fantastic carvings outside the aisles and tower, and a 15th century chancel with good sedilia.

A423 (often busy) on to Deddington ($2\frac{1}{2}$ miles).

Deddington is a former market town with attractive ironstone houses and inns. The wide 14th century Church (to the east on B4031) retains the 13th century sedilia and piscina, and has a 15th century north porch and tower rebuilt after its collapse in 1634. Farther east are the earthworks of the Castle in which Piers Gaveston, the favourite of Edward II, was seized by the Earl of Warwick in 1312.

A423 on for 2 miles, then by an unclassified road (left) and another road (right, in $\frac{1}{2}$ mile, before North Aston) to Steeple Aston (2 miles more).

Steeple Aston is a large village of limestone houses whose restored Church contains an 18th century monument with figures sculptured by Peter Scheemakers.

Unclassified road on from Steeple Aston, crossing B4030 to the entrance to Rousham House ($1\frac{1}{2}$ miles).

Rousham House (admission June-August, Wednesdays and Bank Holidays, 2 to 6; gardens also on Sundays) was built about 1635 and enlarged in 1738-41 by two wings designed by William Kent, who also redecorated part of the interior and laid out the gardens reaching down to the Cherwell, the only unspoilt example of his landscape gardening. The house, further extended by a north front in 1877, has painted ceilings, good portraits, etc., and a chain and jewel given by Charles I to Sir Charles Cottrell, whose family has held the estate since 1540.

Unclassified road back, then B4030 (right) to Middleton Stoney ($4\frac{1}{2}$ miles), then A43 (right) to Weston-on-the-Green (3 miles).

Weston-on-the-Green has a fine house, Weston Manor, partly of the 15th century and now a hotel.

A43 on for $4\frac{1}{2}$ miles, to join A423 at the south end of Kidlington ($1\frac{1}{2}$ miles). A423 south to Oxford ($4\frac{1}{2}$ miles), which is entered by Banbury Road and St. Giles.

36

6. The Vale of Aylesbury : South-Western Part

This tour, starting from the interesting old market and county town of Aylesbury, explores the southern part of the rich, fertile Vale of Aylesbury, the valley of the river Thame, a tributary of the Thames. It keeps mainly to the minor roads, running through quiet and unspoilt country, and takes in some charming villages, among them Long Crendon, Brill on its hilltop, Islip and Aynho; delightful towns such as Thame, Bicester, Brackley and Buckingham; fine houses like Hartwell House, Wotton Underwood, Aynhoe House and Ascott (at Wing); and a variety of characteristic churches, of which the most notable are those at Stewkley and Wing; and includes also the famous grounds of Stowe School.

Aylesbury, the county and assize town of Buckinghamshire, lies in the centre of the Vale of Aylesbury. An important agricultural centre with a large cattle market, and noted for its dairy produce and ducks, it is now partly surrounded by a small industrial belt with engineering and printing works. In the irregularly-shaped Market Place are statues of the politicians, John Hampden and Lord Beaconsfield. On the south side is the 18th century County Hall, preserving its original court, and farther south are the prominent fortress-like County Offices, opened in 1966. Around the square are some of the town's notable old inns: the Bell, largely of the 18th century; the Bull's Head, partly of the 15th century; and the mid-15th century King's Head, which has contemporary stained glass; and in the streets leading northward to the parish church are many prosperous 18th century houses. The County Museum (admission weekdays, 9.30 to 12.30 and 1.30 to 5), in Church Street, has good collections of Buckinghamshire antiquities, costumes and natural history. St. Mary's Church is a large building, mainly of the 13th century, with 15th century additions, but grossly over-restored. It has a massive central tower and a richly-sculptured Norman font of a distinctive local type; and in the south transept is a rare 15th century vestment press.

A418, leaving Aylesbury (Market Place) on the west by Friarage Road and Oxford Road, to Hartwell (2 miles).

Hartwell has an early-Gothic Revival Church (by Henry Keene, 1755), now unhappily in ruins, in the grounds of Hartwell House (admission early May to late July, Wednesdays and Spring Bank Holiday Saturdays, Sundays and Mondays, 2 to 6; gardens only, on Wednesdays in September), a large Jacobean mansion remodelled in the 18th century (partly by Keene). Occupied by the exiled Louis XVIII of France in 1807-14, it was restored after a fire in 1963 and is occupied by the House of Citizenship, a training college for girls.

A418 on to Dinton (on the left).

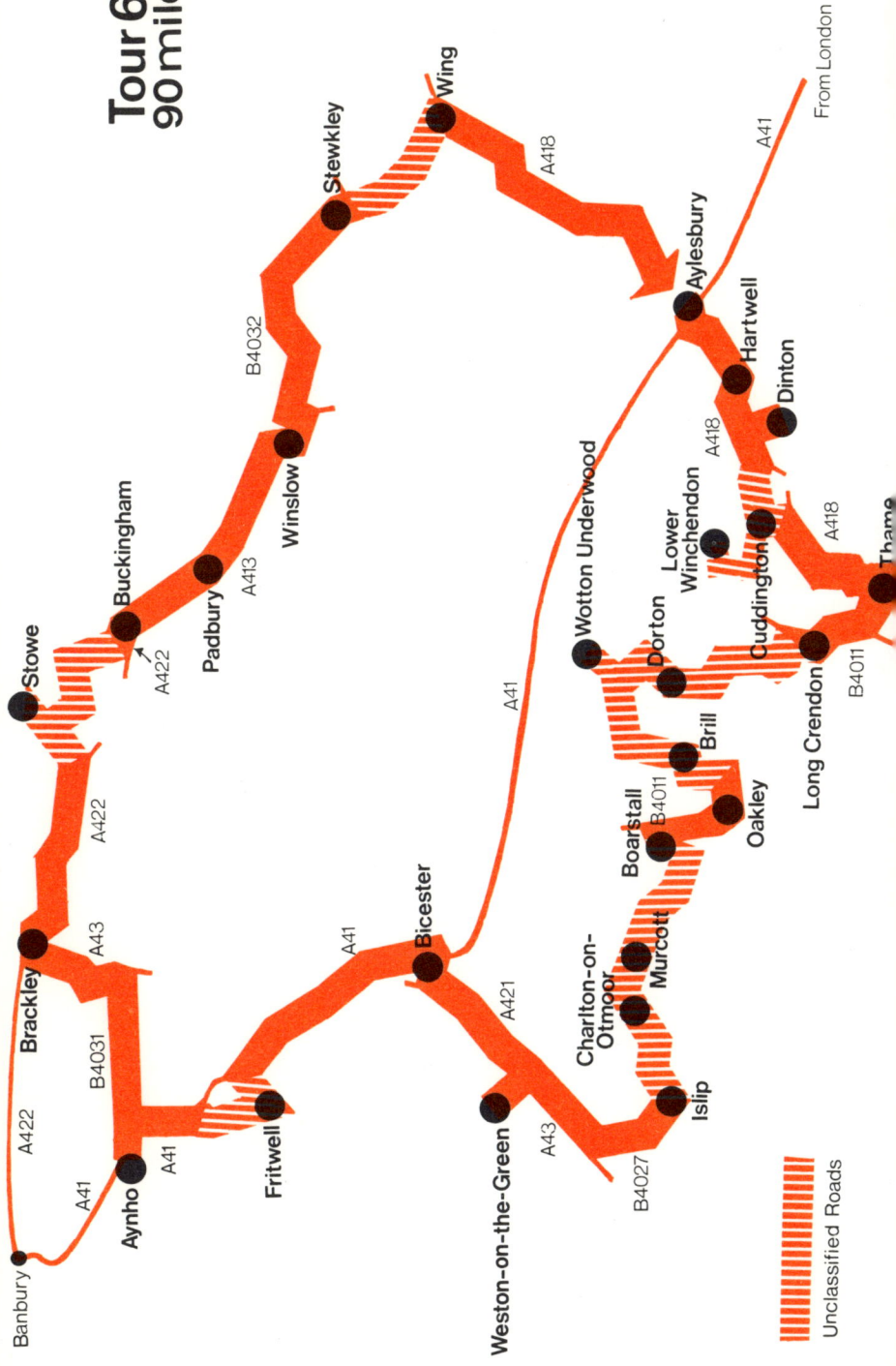

Tour 6
90 miles

N

From London

A41

Wing

A418

Stewkley

Aylesbury

B4032

Hartwell

Dinton

Winslow

A418

Buckingham

Lower
Winchendon

Padbury

A413

Wotton Underwood

Cuddington

A418

Thame

Stowe

Dorton

A422

A41

Brill

Long Crendon

B4011

A422

Boarstall

Oakley

A43

B4011

Brackley

Bicester

Murcott

B4031

A41

Charlton-on-
Otmoor

A422

A41

A421

Islip

Aynho

A41

Fritwell

Weston-on-the-Green

A43

Banbury

B4027

Unclassified Roads

Dinton has a rambling Manor House, partly medieval, and a 13th and 15th century Church with an elaborate Norman doorway.

Unclassified road (right) through Cuddington (2 miles), then right and right again to Lower Winchendon ($1\frac{1}{2}$ miles). [A418, see below, goes on direct to Thame.]

Lower Winchendon is a village in the quiet valley of Thame. Nether Winchendon House (admission Thursdays in May-August, and Easter, Spring and Summer Bank Holidays, 2 to 6), the home of Sir Francis Bernard, governor of New Jersey and Massachusetts in 1761, is a Tudor building enlarged and Gothicised in about 1780.

Unclassified road back to Cuddington (see above), then by another road (right) for $\frac{1}{2}$ mile and A418 (right again) to Thame (4 miles farther).

Thame is a market town with a pleasing variety of 17th-18th century brick and timber-framed houses and inns in its exceptionally wide main street. The large 13th-15th century Church, in the Long Crendon road (see below), has late medieval screens, stalls and brasses. In the chancel is the splendid 16th century tomb of John, Lord Williams, who founded the Grammar School where John Hampden was educated. The original building of 1570 still stands, to the south, and near by is a fine brick and timber tithe-barn.

A418 on (west) from the High Street, then B4011 (right), passing the church and crossing the Thame, to Long Crendon (2 miles).

Long Crendon is a large village with many thatched stone and other attractive old houses. A road on the left passes the 15th century gatehouse of the Manor House, which is of the 15th-16th centuries and partly timber framed. In a road to the right is the interesting 13th-15th century Church, with the fine 17th century monument of Sir John Dormer in the south transept. Close by is the long timber-framed Courthouse, of the 14th or 15th century and probably once a wool staple hall.

Unclassified road right from B4011, towards the church, then left via Chilton to Dorton ($4\frac{1}{2}$ miles).

Dorton has a large Jacobean brick mansion, altered in the late-18th century and now a school.

Unclassified road on for $\frac{1}{2}$ mile, then left and in $\frac{1}{2}$ mile more right for Wotton Underwood ($\frac{1}{2}$ mile farther).

Wotton Underwood is a secluded hamlet with an over-restored Church which contains a rare columbarium (of about 1800) and monuments of the Grenvilles, Dukes of Buckingham, who lived near by at the stately Wotton House (admission June-September, Wednesdays, 2 to 6). Built in 1704-14 by an unknown architect, this was reconstructed internally with classic grace (after a fire in 1820) by Sir John Soane. The park was the first individual piece of landscaping by ‘ Capability ’ Brown.

Unclassified road back to reach the Dorton road, then right to Brill (3 miles).

Brill is a brick-built village beautifully situated on the top of an isolated hill rising from the Vale, with charming views towards the Chiltern Hills.

Unclassified road (right; i.e. south-west) to Oakley ($1\frac{1}{2}$ miles), then B4011 (right) for $1\frac{1}{2}$ miles and by an unclassified road (left) to Boarstall ($\frac{1}{2}$ mile).

Boarstall has a moated gatehouse of the 14th-17th centuries, the only remaining part of a fortified manor house.

Unclassified road on, bearing right twice and left to Murcott, and thence to Charlton-on-Otmoor ($4\frac{1}{2}$ miles).

Charlton-on-Otmoor is a limestone village on the north edge of Ot Moor, a curious flat round-shaped tract of land, once a marsh. The Church, mainly of the 14th century, has a well-preserved rood-screen and loft of about 1500, surmounted by a cross-garland of box leaves.

Unclassified road on via Oddington to Islip (3 miles).

Islip (see also Tour 5) is a charming village of limestone cottages, at the junction of the river Ray with the Cherwell.

B4027 (right) for 1 mile, then A43 (right again) to Weston-on-the-Green ($1\frac{1}{2}$ miles; to the left, on Tour 5) and A421 on, following the course of the Roman Akeman Street, to Bicester ($4\frac{1}{2}$ miles farther; on the right).

Bicester is an agricultural town and a noted hunting centre, with old houses around the market place. The restored Church, partly Saxon, has 13th-14th century nave arcades and the Norman arches of a vanished tower.

A41 north (crossing A421 and A43), then by an unclassified road (left) to Fritwell (7 miles).

Fritwell is a pleasant limestone village with a delightful Jacobean manor house. The restored 12th-15th century Church is dedicated (unusually) to St. Olaf, the patron saint of Norway.

Unclassified road (right; i.e. north), rejoining A41 for Aynho (3 miles).

Aynho is a charming village on a hill above the Cherwell, remarkable especially for the apricots growing on its cottage walls. Aynhoe Park (admission May-September, Wednesdays and Thursdays, 2 to 5), a fine 17th century house altered by Thomas Archer in 1707-14 and Sir John Soane in 1802, is now a home of the Mutual Households Association.

A41 back for $\frac{1}{2}$ mile, then B4031 on through Croughton for $3\frac{1}{2}$ miles and A43 (left) to Brackley ($2\frac{1}{2}$ miles).

Brackley is a delightful stone-built market town with a wide High Street in which the Town Hall, built in 1707, has been attributed to Wren. Magdalen College School, established in 1548, incorporates the restored chapel of St. James's Hospital, an almshouse

founded about 1150. On the chapel are niches containing (unusually) their original statues, and others are to be seen on the fine 13th century tower of St. Peter's Church, outside the town to the north-east.

A422 east via Westbury for over 4½ miles, then by an unclassified road (left) to the grounds of Stowe (nearly 1 mile).

Stowe, long the palatial seat of the Temples, Dukes of Buckingham, has been since 1923 a well-known public school. Begun about 1718 for Sir Richard Temple, Lord Cobham, it has a north portico attributed to Vanbrugh and a fine south front added by Robert Adam in 1774. The beautiful grounds (admission Good Friday to Easter Monday and for a fortnight in August, 2 to 6.30), laid out after 1713, are notable for their classical temples, etc., by Vanbrugh, Gibbs and Kent.

Unclassified road east from the entrance to the Stowe grounds, then left and right, through an avenue of elms (1½ miles long in all), to join A422 at Buckingham (3 miles).

Buckingham, once the county town, is an old agricultural centre on the Great Ouse, with several fine houses. In the Market Square is the 18th century Town Hall; at the east end of the adjoining Market Hill is the Old Gaol, built in 1758, and near the west corner of the Hill is a Chantry Chapel (key at No. 4, West Street), rebuilt in 1475, but retaining a Norman doorway. The Church, on a hill to the south, was built in 1781, but greatly altered in 1865 by Sir Gilbert Scott.

A413 south-east from the Market Place, via Padbury, to Winslow (6 miles).

Winslow is an attractive small town with old houses around the Market Square. Winslow Hall, passed on A413 (below), is a stately house of 1700, confidently ascribed to Sir Christopher Wren.

A413 on for ½ mile, then B4032 (left) via Swanbourne to Stewkley (6½ miles).

Stewkley is a village with a long street of old cottages and an unspoilt and richly-decorated late-Norman Church.

Unclassified road on, beyond the church, to Wing (3 miles).

Wing is a large village remarkable for its complete Saxon Church, with its original nave and chancel arches, apse and crypt, and notable 16th-17th century monuments. Ascott (admission April-September, Wednesdays, Saturdays and Bank Holiday Mondays, 2 to 6; also certain Sundays in July and August), ½ mile east near the Leighton Buzzard road (A418), is a house rebuilt after 1873 for the Rothschilds, the banker family, and contains a superb collection of furniture, porcelain and paintings. The charming grounds command a view towards the Chilterns.

A418 south-west to Aylesbury (7 miles).

Tour 7
91 miles

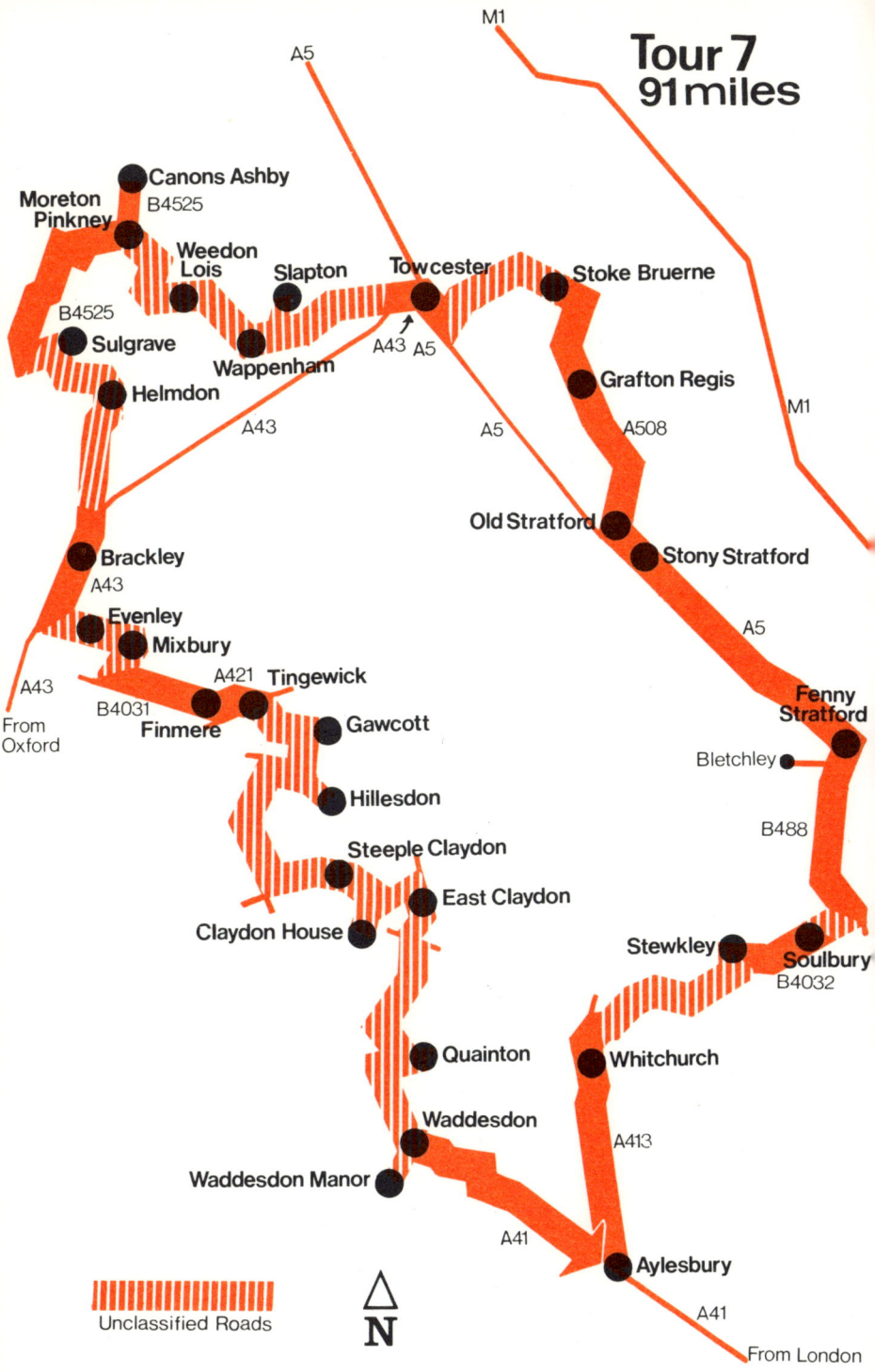

M1

A5

Canons Ashby

Moreton Pinkney

B4525

Weedon Lois

Slapton

Towcester

Stoke Bruerne

B4525

Sulgrave

Wappenham

A43 A5

Grafton Regis

Helmdon

A43

A5

A508

M1

Old Stratford

Stony Stratford

Brackley

A43

Evenley

Mixbury

A421

Tingewick

A5

From Oxford

A43

B4031

Finmere

Gawcott

Fenny Stratford

Hillesdon

Bletchley

Steeple Claydon

B488

East Claydon

Claydon House

Stewkley

Soulbury

B4032

Quainton

Whitchurch

Waddesdon

A413

Waddesdon Manor

A41

Aylesbury

From London

Unclassified Roads

N

7. The Vale of Aylesbury : North-Eastern Part

This tour, like the previous one, starts at Aylesbury and it covers the northern part of the Vale of Aylesbury and part of the adjacent valley of the Great Ouse and its tributaries. Like Tour 6, too, it keeps to unclassified and little-used roads as far as possible, and it likewise takes in attractive villages, interesting old towns (such as Fenny and Stony Stratford, Towcester and Brackley), and two houses of outstanding interest—Claydon House and Waddesdon Manor—as well as some characteristic churches and places of such diverse interest as the Canal Museum and Stoke Bruerne and the home of George Washington's ancestors at Sulgrave.

Aylesbury is described in Tour 6 (page 37).

A413, leaving Aylesbury (Market Place) on the north by Kingsbury Square and Buckingham Street, across the Thame to Hardwick and thence to Whitchurch (4½ miles).

Whitchurch is a village among the rich meadows of the Vale, with many attractive houses and an unspoilt 14th century Church.

A413 on for 1½ miles, then by an unclassified road (right) via Dunton to Stewkley (4 miles more).

Stewkley has a long village street with many old houses and an untouched late-Norman Church, richly decorated.

B4032 (right) to Soulbury (2 miles), then by an unclassified road to Three Locks (1 mile), in the Ouzel valley; then B488 (left again) via Stoke Hammond to Fenny Stratford (4 miles).

Fenny Stratford stands on the Ouzel, a tributary of the Great Ouse, and on the course of the Roman road of Watling Street, which ran from London to Chester. The 'Fenny Poppers' are tiny cannon that are fired in the churchyard at Martinmas (11th November) in honour of Browne Willis, the antiquary, who in 1730 rebuilt the Church. This has a remarkable panelled ceiling, with shields of arms, in the north aisle, but it was greatly enlarged in an ornate Gothic style in 1866. Fenny Stratford is adjoined on the west by Bletchley, a railway centre and an expanding town with numerous engineering and other works

A5 north-west, following the straight course of Watling Street, to Stony Stratford (7 miles).

Stony Stratford is an old coaching town with 18th century houses and inns. The tales interchanged by travellers at the two principal hotels (the Cock and the Bull) are said to have been the foundation of the phrase " a cock and bull story ". [B4033, leading south-west from the cross-roads, passes the end of a road (right) to Passenham (1 mile), a hamlet on the Ouse which has a church with a 13th century tower and nave, and a chancel rebuilt in 1626, when the unusual woodwork was introduced and the wall paintings were executed. The road goes to A422, which runs north to Old Stratford (1½ miles).]

A5 on from Stony Stratford over the Ouse to Old Stratford (1 mile), then A508 (right) to Grafton Regis (4 miles).

Grafton Regis is a village of thatched stone cottages on a hill above the Tove, another tributary of the Ouse. In the 14th-15th century Church Edward IV was married in 1464 to Elizabeth Woodville, whom he is supposed to have met under the Queen's Oak, to the south-west near the A5 at the edge of Whittlewood Forest.

A508 on, crossing the Grand Union Canal, then by an unclassified road (left) to Stoke Bruerne ($2\frac{1}{2}$ miles).

Stoke Bruerne, pleasantly situated on the canal, with a hump-backed bridge, a canalside inn and a picturesque lock, has an interesting Waterways Museum (admission daily, 10 to 12.30, 2 to 5 and 6 to 8). Blisworth Tunnel, opening to the north of the village, is the longest canal tunnel in England ($1\frac{3}{4}$ miles).

Unclassified road, recrossing the canal, to Shutlanger (1 mile) and thence across the Tove for $2\frac{1}{2}$ miles more; then A5 (right), skirting the park of Easton Neston, to Towcester ($1\frac{1}{2}$ miles).

Towcester is a small town on the Tove, with a charming old inn (the Saracen's Head) and other ironstone houses. The 13th-15th century Church contains the fine tomb of Archdeacon Sponne, a 15th century benefactor, and an 18th century organ of Continental make, brought from Fonthill Abbey, in Wiltshire. Easton Neston, whose gardens (reached from A43, to the north) are open occasionally, is a classical house of the early 18th century designed by Nicholas Hawksmoor for the Fermor family, whose monuments are in the 15th century church near by.

A43 west from Towcester for $\frac{1}{2}$ mile, then by an unclassified road (right) via Abthorpe to Slapton (3 miles; on the right).

Slapton, on a slope above the Tove, has a secluded 13th-14th century Church with a wealth of 14th century wall paintings.

Unclassified road on (continuing the road west from Towcester) to Wappenham (1 mile).

Wappenham has a plain 13th and 15th century Church and a Vicarage built by Sir Gilbert Scott for his father, Rev. Thomas Scott, who was rector here. The more direct road going on westward to Sulgrave ($5\frac{1}{2}$ miles; see below), via Helmdon, passes near Astwell Castle ($1\frac{1}{2}$ miles), a fortified 15th century manor house.

Unclassified road north from Wappenham church, crossing the Tove to Weedon Lois ($2\frac{1}{2}$ miles) and thence to Weston ($\frac{1}{2}$ mile).

Weedon Lois has a Church, mostly of the 14th century, with a 15th century stone pulpit. In the churchyard extension to the east is the grave of Edith Sitwell, the poet, who died in 1965, and a memorial to her, with sculpture by Henry Moore, is to be placed here. Weston has a hall mainly of the 17th-18th centuries.

Unclassified road on, branching right, then left, to Moreton Pinkney (2 miles); thence B4525 (right) to Canons Ashby (1 mile).

Canons Ashby has a 16th century house (long the home of the Dryden family) enlarged in the early-18th century, and a Church with a finely-sculptured 13th century doorway, formerly the church of an Augustinian priory.

B4525 back through Moreton Pinkney and on for $3\frac{1}{2}$ miles more, then by an unclassified road (left) to Sulgrave ($\frac{1}{2}$ mile).

Sulgrave is a pleasant limestone village, famous as the home of the Washington family, ancestors of the President, from 1539 until 1610. In the south aisle of the restored Church is the brass of Lawrence Washington, the seventh ancestor in direct ascent of George Washington, and the 17th century Washington pew. Sulgrave Manor (admission daily, except Wednesdays, 10.30 to 1 and 2 to 4 or, in April-September, to 5.30), at the east end of the village, was bought and rebuilt about 1560 by Lawrence Washington, a successful wool-merchant of Northampton. The house was purchased by a trust in 1914, the centenary of the Treaty of Ghent, marking a century of peace between Britain and the United States, and opened in 1921 as a Washington Museum, and it contains furniture, etc., contemporary with the great President, including his chair from Mount Vernon, as well as relics and portraits of him. On the south porch are the Washington arms, generally regarded as the origin of the ' Stars and Stripes '.

Unclassified road south-east from the church to Helmdon (3 miles), then south to join A43 in $3\frac{1}{2}$ miles, about 1 mile short of Brackley.

Brackley is described in Tour 6 (page 40).

A43 on for 1 mile, then by an unclassified road (left) to Evenley ($\frac{1}{2}$ mile).

Evenley has rows of cottages attractively arranged round a green, at the entrance to Evenley Park.

Unclassified road on through Mixbury for 2 miles, then B4031 (left) to Finmere ($2\frac{1}{2}$ miles) and A421 on to Tingewick (1 mile).

Tingewick has a Church, partly of about 1200, with memorials to Admiral Lord Keyes, the first Chief of Combined Operations (who died in 1945), and his son, Lt.-Col. Geoffrey Keyes (killed in 1941), who lived at Tingewick House. A minor road to the north, crossing the Ouse, leads to Water Stratford (1 mile), which has a small church with fine Norman sculpture on its doorways.

Unclassified road south-east from Tingewick to Gawcott ($1\frac{1}{2}$ miles).

Gawcott is a pleasing village with brick and stone houses. The classical Church was designed for himself in 1827 by Thomas Scott, rector for 27 years (until he moved to Wappenham in 1833) and the father of Sir George Gilbert Scott, the apostle of Victorian Gothic, who was born here in 1811.

Unclassified road on, forking left in $\frac{1}{2}$ mile, to Hillesdon (2 miles).

Hillesdon is a remote hamlet on a low hill, with a complete 15th century Church which has many notable features, including the fine fan-vaulted porch, the unusual staircase-tower with its open crown, and the stone panelling and rows of carved angels in the chancel.

Unclassified road back and left, then left again (in $1\frac{1}{2}$ miles), crossing a tributary of the Ouse, and left yet again (in 2 miles more) to the large village of Steeple Claydon ($1\frac{1}{2}$ miles); then right and left here to pass the entrance to Claydon House at Middle Claydon ($1\frac{1}{2}$ miles farther).

Claydon House (admission March-October, Tuesday to Sunday and Bank Holiday Mondays, 2 to 6; closed Tuesdays after Bank Holidays; November-February, by appointment only), the seat of the Verney family, was partly built about 1760-80 by a carpenter-contractor named Lightfoot, who was responsible also for the decoration of the most amazing suite of rococo rooms in England, with much exuberant wood carving. On the first floor are an astounding 'Chinese' room and many memorials of Florence Nightingale, who often visited her sister here. Concerts (arranged by the National Trust) are given in summer in the Saloon, which has excellent acoustics. In the Church close by is the fine monument of Sir Edmund Verney, who fell at the Battle of Edgehill in 1642.

Unclassified on and right to East Claydon (2 miles), then right to Botolph Claydon (1 mile); then left here and by the third road on the left to Quainton (3 miles more).

Quainton is a large village with a pleasant green and attractive 17th century almshouses, well situated on the south slope of Quainton Hill, with a view towards the Chilterns. The 14th-15th century Church, at the east end, has many fine brasses and monuments.

Unclassified road south, crossing the railway at Quainton Road station, then left to Waddesdon ($2\frac{1}{2}$ miles), where the entrance to Waddesdon Manor is to the right, along A41.

Waddesdon Manor (admission late March to late October, Wednesday to Sunday, 2 to 6; Bank Holiday Mondays, 11 to 6; on Fridays the charge is raised, but additional rooms are open), dramatically placed on the top of a hill enclosed by beautiful woods, is an imposing mansion in the style of a French château, built in 1874-80 by a French architect, H.-A. Destailleur, for Baron Ferdinand de Rothschild, the banker. The stately rooms are full of artistic treasures gathered by the Rothschilds, mostly French and of the 18th century, and including paintings, tapestries, carpets, furniture and a great range of porcelain, as well as panelling from noble Parisian houses. The village of Waddesdon has many contemporary houses built under the Rothschild patronage.

A41 east, crossing the Thame, to Aylesbury ($5\frac{1}{2}$ miles).

8. The Great Ouse Valley and the Bedfordshire Uplands

Starting from Dunstable, an old market town with a fine priory church below the escarpment of the Chiltern Hills, and easily reached by the M1 Motorway (about 2 miles east), this tour explores the wide vale of the Great Ouse, in effect a northern extension of the Vale of Aylesbury. Keeping mainly to minor roads, it takes in the thriving county and industrial town of Bedford, several smaller but interesting towns—Fenny Stratford, Newport Pagnell, Olney and Ampthill—some charming villages, such as Weston Underwood, Turvey and Stevington, and various attractive churches. Beyond Elstow, famous for its associations with John Bunyan, it traverses a line of sandstone hills and visits two widely differing houses, the ruined Jacobean mansion of Houghton Hall and the splendid 18th century house of Woburn Abbey.

Dunstable is mainly a residential town, but has an industrial quarter on the east, towards Luton. The Parish Church, though restored, preserves the grand Norman nave and west portal and the 13th century tower and west front of an Augustinian priory founded in 1131 by Henry I. Near the northern section of the High Street is the fine Civic Centre, completed in 1964, with a good concert hall. Dunstable Downs, which rise to the south, are the northernmost extremity of the main stretch of the Chiltern Hills,

B489 west from the cross-roads for 1 mile, then by an unclassified road (right) to Totternhoe (1 mile).

Totternhoe is a long village on an outlying knoll facing the Dunstable Downs. The 14th-16th century Church, at the south end, is built almost entirely of chalk-stone from the quarries for which the village was famous during the Middle Ages.

Unclassified road, passing the church, then right for Eaton Bray (1½ miles).

Eaton Bray has a Church with fine 13th century ironwork decoration on the south door, by Thomas of Leighton (Buzzard), a noted smith who worked in Westminster Abbey, and 13th century nave arcades of Totternhoe chalk, with well-carved capitals.

Unclassified road left, over ¼ mile beyond the church, to Billington (2½ miles), then B486 (right) to Leighton Buzzard (2 miles).

Leighton Buzzard, on the Ouzel (a tributary of the Ouse), is an old market town noted for its sand, used in tile-making. In the wide High Street is a pentagonal Market Cross of about 1400. The Church, largely of the 13th century, has an imposing tower and spire, 191 feet high, and ironwork by Thomas of Leighton. Inside are a rare medieval eagle lectern of wood, 15th century monastic stalls, and 24 characteristic Victorian stained glass windows by C. E. Kempe.

Tour 8
73 miles

N

From Northampton

Weston Underwood — A509
Olney — B565
Ravenstone
Tyringham
Gayhurst — A50
M1
Newport Pagnell
A50
Broughton
Milton Keynes
A5
Simpson
Fenny Stratford
B488
A5
Linslade — A418
Leighton Buzzard
B486
Billington
Eaton Bray

Turvey — A428
Stevington
Oakley
Clapham — A6
Bedford
Elstow — A6
Wilshamstead
Houghton Conquest
A418
Houghton House
Ampthill
Ridgmont — A418
Woburn
Woburn Abbey
A50
Milton Bryan
A5120
Toddington
Chalgrave
Houghton Regis
M1
Totternhoe
A5
Dunstable
B489 — A505
Luton
M1
From London

|||||||||| Unclassified Roads

A418 over the Ouzel to Linslade ($\frac{1}{2}$ mile), then B488 (right) through the valley to Fenny Stratford (6$\frac{1}{2}$ miles).

Fenny Stratford is described in Tour 7 (page 43).

B488 on over A5 to Simpson (1$\frac{1}{2}$ miles), then by an unclassified road (right), over the Ouzel to Walton ($\frac{1}{2}$ mile), then left to Milton Keynes (2 miles).

Milton Keynes, a village with a 14th century Church, is to give its name to a 'new city' of some 250,000 inhabitants which is to extend from the M1 Motorway over the A5.

Unclassified road (right) to join A50 short of Broughton (1 mile), then over the M1 to Newport Pagnell (3 miles).

Newport Pagnell, at the junction of the Ouzel with the Great Ouse, has noted motor-engineering works, but is mainly an agricultural town. The spacious 14th-15th century Church is much restored.

A50 on through Gayhurst (2$\frac{1}{2}$ miles), then by an unclassified road (right), branching right and left for Ravenstone (3 miles more).

Ravenstone has thatched stone cottages and a Church with good 17th century woodwork and the dignified monument of Lord Chancellor Finch, 1st Earl of Nottingham.

Unclassified road (right) to Weston Underwood (1$\frac{1}{2}$ miles).

Weston Underwood is a delightful village of limestone houses, many of them of the 18th century, including one in which the poet, William Cowper (see below), lived in 1786-95.

Unclassified road on to Olney (1$\frac{1}{2}$ miles).

Olney, on the Great Ouse, is a pleasant small stone-built town making footwear. In the Market Place is a large 17th century brick house, now the Cowper Memorial Museum (admission week-days, 10 to 5), where William Cowper lived in 1767-86, here writing 'John Gilpin' and 'The Task'. The 14th century Church, to the south, has a fine tower and spire, 185 feet high. A Pancake Race takes place in Olney on Shrove Tuesday, in competition with the women of Liberal (Kansas), U.S.A.

A509 north for over $\frac{1}{2}$ mile, then B565 (right) for nearly 2$\frac{1}{2}$ miles and A428 (right again) to Turvey (1 mile).

Turvey, attractively situated on the Ouse, is a model village with a variety of stone-built houses. The restored Church has 13th century ironwork by Thomas of Leighton, a painted Crucifixion of the 14th century and fine monuments of the Mordaunt family.

A428 on for 2$\frac{1}{2}$ miles, then by an unclassified road (left) to Stevington (1$\frac{1}{2}$ miles).

Stevington a charming village with thatched and whitewashed cottages and a medieval market cross. The Church, near the Ouse, has a partly Saxon tower and notable 13th century arcades. An

18th century post-mill, south of the Oakley road, was restored in 1951 as a memorial to John Bunyan.

Unclassified road (right) for $1\frac{1}{2}$ miles, then left, crossing the river, to Oakley ($\frac{1}{2}$ mile); then right to join A6 in 1 mile, $\frac{1}{2}$ mile short of Clapham.

Clapham, a growing village on the Ouse, has a Church mostly rebuilt in 1861 but with a tall and fine Saxon tower.

A6 on to Bedford ($2\frac{1}{2}$ miles).

Bedford, famous for its associations with John Bunyan, is a busy county and assize town and an industrial centre, with numerous engineering and other works, and is also a popular boating resort and an educational centre. Near St. Peter's Church, which has a Saxon or early-Norman tower and a Norman porch, at the north end of High Street, is a statue of Bunyan, " facing where stood his jail ". John Bunyan moved to Bedford from Elstow (see below) in 1655 and began preaching in the following year; arrested in 1660, he was confined to prison almost continuously for twelve years. To the north are the 19th century buildings of Bedford School, one of the four schools administered under the Harpur Trust, founded by Sir William Harpur in 1552. In Mill Street, on the left of High Street, is the Bunyan Meeting, built in 1849 on the site of the chapel where Bunyan was minister from 1672 until his death in 1688. The Bunyan Museum (admission Tuesday-Friday, 10 to 12 and 2.30 to 4.30) adjoining contains many personal mementoes. High Street goes on past the central St. Paul's Square, with a fine statue of John Howard, the prison reformer, and the restored 14th-15th century Parish Church, which contains the brass of Sir William Harpur and a 15th century stone pulpit. The Town Bridge, crossing the Great Ouse to St. Mary's Church, which has an early-Norman tower, replaces the 13th century bridge on which stood the Town Gaol, where Bunyan was imprisoned in 1675-6 and wrote the first part of the *Pilgrim's Progress*. The Embankment, leading east from the bridge, passes the interesting Bedford Museum (admission weekdays 11 to 5, Sundays 2 to 5), with local antiquities and ' bygones ', and the grounds of Castle Close, which now contain the Cecil Higgins Art Gallery (admission weekdays 11 to 6 or dusk, Sundays from 2.30), an excellent collection of porcelain, glass, furniture and English water-colours.

A6 on, beyond the Ouse, to Elstow ($1\frac{1}{2}$ miles).

Elstow was the early home of John Bunyan, who was born near by in 1628. It was on the village green that, while playing tipcat one Sunday afternoon, he was " put to an exceeding maze " by a vision that led to his conversion. The late-15th century timber-framed Moot Hall here, formerly the meeting-place and school of the Independent congregation that Bunyan joined, is now a museum of English 17th-century life and of traditions connected with Bunyan (admission Tuesday-Saturday, 11 to 1 and 2 to 5; Sundays, 2.30 to 5.30). The much-restored Church, near by, has a detached 15th

century tower and incorporates the Norman and 13th century nave of a Benedictine nunnery. It contains the 15th century font at which Bunyan was baptized and the rare brass of an abbess.

A6 on via Wilshamstead for 4 miles, then by an unclassified road (right) to Houghton Conquest ($1\frac{1}{2}$ miles).

Houghton Conquest is a pleasant village which has a 14th-15th century Church with 15th century wall paintings and brasses.

Unclassified road on for 1 mile, then A418 (left), passing the entrance to Houghton House ($1\frac{1}{2}$ miles; see below), to Ampthill ($\frac{1}{2}$ mile).

Ampthill, on the range of greensand hills that crosses Bedfordshire, is a delightful market town with 18th century houses and inns. The Church, mainly of the 14th and 15th centuries, contains the 17th century monument of Richard Nicholls, the first English governor of New York, who was probably born here. In beautiful grounds skirted by the Woburn road (see below) is Ampthill Park, a fine late-17th century house, now a Cheshire Home for the incurably sick. Houghton House was built about 1615 for the Countess of Pembroke, sister of Sir Philip Sidney, and altered soon afterwards, perhaps by Inigo Jones, but was dismantled in 1794.

A418 west from the cross-roads, along the greensand ridge to Ridgmont, and then, alongside the wall of Woburn Abbey Park, to Woburn ($6\frac{1}{4}$ miles).

Woburn is a delightful small town on the wooded greensand uplands, with many charming 18th century houses. From it, a drive leads to Woburn Abbey (admission daily; April-October, 11.30 to 5, Sundays in June-August to 7; November-March, 1.30 to 4; to the park from 11 or 12.30), the principal seat of the Russell family (Dukes of Bedford), who have been here since 1548. The stately house was mainly built in 1747-61 by Henry Flitcroft, incorporating a wing of about 1630, and was altered in 1788 by Henry Holland. It has good ceilings and mantelpieces, furniture and silver, and Sèvres and other porcelain, and a fine collection of paintings by Holbein, Van Dyck, Reynolds, Gainsborough and other masters, including 24 views of Venice of Canaletto. The beautifully wooded Park, which is about $9\frac{1}{2}$ miles in circumference, has many amusements but contains also some 2,000 animals and birds, notable among which are the deer (especially the Père David herd, introduced from China but now extinct there), the European and American bison, and the rare herd of wild white cattle.

A50 south, skirting Woburn Park (with a view of the house), for 2 miles, then by an unclassified road (left) to Milton Bryan ($\frac{1}{2}$ mile) and right to Toddington (3 miles).

Toddington is a large village with old houses round a green and a 13th-15th century Church which has a unique 16th century three-storey priest's house attached to the chancel.

A5120 (right) via Houghton Regis to join A5 in $4\frac{1}{2}$ miles and 1 mile short of Dunstable.

Tour 9
99 miles

Unclassified Roads

N

M1

M1

Whipsnade
Whipsnade Zoo
B4506 B4540
B489
Little Gaddesden
Netteden
B486
Piccotts End
Hemel Hempstead
Apsley
A414
A41
Kings Langley
A411
Watford
Bushey
Bushey Heath
A4140
Moor Park
Northwood
A4005
A409
Harrow-on-the-Hill
Sudbury
A404
Harlesden
A5
LONDON
Marble Arch
Shepherd's Bush
A40
Hanger Lane
A406
A40
A40
Northolt Aerodrome
Ruislip
B455
A404
Rickmansworth
Chorleywood
B485
Chenies
Latimer
Chesham
A416
Amersham
A413
Little Missenden
A413
Great Missenden
A4128
Prestwood
Great Hampden
Chequers
B4010
Halton
Wendover
A4011
A41
Tring
Drayton Beauchamp
B488
Ivinghoe
Edlesborough
B4506
Aldbury
Ashridge

9. The Northern Chilterns, with Whipsnade Zoo

This tour explores the northern section of the Chiltern Hills (see Tour 2), with the highest and most beautiful country. It takes an easy and pleasant way out of London, crossing the Colne valley and ascending that of the Chess to Chesham. It then takes in the delightful old town of Amersham, ascends the Misbourne via the quiet villages of Great and Little Missenden, and crosses a well-wooded and secluded reach of the Chilterns to Chenies, week-end home of the Prime Minister, and the charming village of Wendover. The route then follows the Chiltern escarpment through Tring and the interesting villages of Aldbury and Ivinghoe before ascending to Whipsnade, with the popular country zoo of the Zoological Society of London. The return to London is made via the valley of the Gade and Hemel Hempstead, now the nucleus of one of the finest of the New Towns. Those who have time may also take in Watford and Harrow-on-the-Hill, famous for its school, on the way back.

From London (Marble Arch) by Bayswater Road (north of Hyde Park) and Holland Park Avenue (A40) to Shepherd's Bush, then by Wood Lane and the White City Stadium to Hanger Lane (North Circular Road; 7 miles) and on by A40 (Western Avenue) to Northolt Aerodrome (5 miles); then by B455 (right) to Ruislip (2 miles).

Ruislip is a favourite residential district with the nucleus of its old village, with timber-framed houses round the medieval Parish Church, at the north end of High Street. Farther north is the restored 16th century Manor Farm House, which has interesting old weatherboarded barns (one now a public library). Ruislip Lido (see below), a wood-fringed reservoir, has facilities for bathing, sailing and water ski-ing.

B455 on, passing west of Ruislip Lido, to Northwood (3 miles), then A404 (left) to Batchworth Heath (1 mile), at the entrance to Moor Park.

Northwood is another favoured residential district, in a hilly situation. Moor Park (admission Mondays, except Bank Holidays, 2 to 6, or by previous arrangement), now a golf-club house, is a splendid classical mansion rebuilt in 1720 by Sir James Thornhill and Giacomo Leoni, with elaborate interior decoration.

A404 on, descending to Rickmansworth (1½ miles).

Rickmansworth, a largely residential town on the Colne, has some old houses near the church. William Penn, the founder of Pennsylvania, lived for five years after his marriage in 1644 at Basing House (now the council offices) in the High Street. The Aquadrome, to the west, a reservoir built to serve the Grand Union Canal, is a centre for sailing, bathing and water ski-ing.

A404 on through Chorleywood (2 miles), then B485 (right) to Chenies (1½ miles) and thence to Latimer (1 mile; on the right).

53

Chenies is a model village with houses of about 1850, in the pleasant Chess valley. An avenue leads to the enlarged Tudor Manor House, long the seat of the Russell family, Dukes of Bedford, whose extensive and splendid series of monuments are in the north chapel of the renewed 15th-16th century Church. At Latimer, a pretty village in the Chess valley, the Joint Services' Staff College occupies Latimer House, an elaborate building of 1863.

B485 on up the valley to Chesham (4 miles).

Chesham, though largely a residential town, has old-established woodenware and brush-making industries. Around the restored 13th-15th century Church is a nucleus of old houses, among them The Bury of 1712.

A416 south, crossing a ridge to the Misbourne valley, then A404 (right) to Amersham (3 miles).

Amersham is an enchanting old agricultural town with a long main street containing many 17th-18th century houses and inns. In the centre is the brick Town Hall of 1682, with an open market space below. The Victorianised Church has many brasses and fine monuments, mostly of the Drake family, who lived at Shardeloes, an 18th century house, chiefly an early work of Robert Adam, in a verdant park with a lake.

A413 on up the valley, then by an unclassified road (left) to Little Missenden (3 miles).

Little Missenden is an attractive village whose interesting Church is basically Saxon, but was altered in the 13th-15th centuries and is noted for its variety of medieval wall paintings.

A413 on again, up the Misbourne, then an unclassified road (left) to Great Missenden (2 miles).

Great Missenden is another attractive village in the beautiful Chiltern valley. Missenden Abbey, now an adult education college, is an 18th century Gothic mansion incorporating a few remains of a house of Arrouaisian canons founded in 1133.

A4128 (left), ascending on to the Chiltern plateau at Prestwood (2 miles), then by an unclassified road (right), passing the Hampden monument (see below), to Great Hampden (1½ miles).

Great Hampden, on the edge of another Chiltern valley, has a restored 14th-15th century Church with a monument to John Hampden, the Parliamentarian statesman, who lived at Hampden House (now a girl's school), Gothicised in the 18th century, but embodying a late-medieval tower. In the grounds to the west is a length of Grim's Ditch, an earthwork of unknown purpose, but possibly Saxon in origin. Beside the road from Prestwood is a stone cross marking the ' parcel of land ' for which Hampden refused to pay the illegal ' ship-money ' tax of 20s., an act which first brought him to public notice.

Unclassified road back, then left, descending into the valley; then left again, under the fine beechwoods of Little Hampden,

branching right at a fork-roads and passing the entrance to Chequers (2½ miles).

Chequers (no admission) is an Elizabethan house enlarged and much altered by Lord Lee of Fareham, who in 1917 presented it to the nation for the use of the Prime Minister. To the east of the park and road rises Coombe Hill (852 feet), the highest point of the Chiltern Hills, commanding a wide view over the Vale of Aylesbury.

Unclassified road on, descending through a gap in the Chiltern escarpment, to Butler's Cross (1 mile), then B4010 (right) to Wendover (1½ miles).

Wendover is a charming village with many 17th and 18th century houses, mostly of brick, delightfully situated at the entrance to another gap in the Chiltern Hills.

A413 and A4011 on past Halton (1½ miles) to Bucklandwharf (2 miles), then A41 (right), following the course of the Roman Akeman Street.

Halton, below the beautifully-wooded escarpment of the Chilterns, has a large R.A.F. station incorporating Halton House, built in 1884 for the Rothschilds, the influential bankers. A road on the left beyond the junction with A41 leads to the hamlet of Drayton Beauchamp, which has a secluded church of the 13th-16th centuries with interesting brasses and stained glass.

A41 on, below the Chilterns, to Tring (1½ miles).

Tring, a market and residential town, has a restored 15th century Church with a finely-sculptured monument of 1707 attributed to Grinling Gibbons. The parish registers contain entries referring to the ancestors of President George Washington. Tring Park, to the south, houses an excellent Zoological Museum (admission weekdays 2 to 5, in winter 1 to 4; Bank Holidays 10 to 12 and 2 to 5; Sundays 2 to 4.30) created by the 2nd Baron Rothschild and now a department of the British Museum (Natural History).

A41 on from the church, then by an unclassified road (left), passing Pendley Manor, to Aldbury (2½ miles).

Aldbury is a charming village with 16th-17th century brick and timber-framed houses spaced round a green with a pond. On Aldbury Common, above the wooded escarpment of the Chilterns, is a tall monument to the 3rd Earl of Bridgwater, the canal-builder, the 'father of inland navigation'. Pendley Manor is a pioneer residential centre of adult education, opened in 1945.

Unclassified road north, under the chalkland escarpment, joining B488 to Ivinghoe (3 miles).

Ivinghoe is an attractive village with brick and timbered houses and a 13th-15th century Church which has richly-foliated capitals to the nave arcades and an elaborate Jacobean pulpit. Pitstone Windmill, to the south, is one of the oldest post-mills in England

(1627). To the east rises Ivinghoe Beacon (700 feet), a distinctive promontory of the Chiltern Hills, crowned by an Iron Age hill-fort and with another wide view over the Vale of Aylesbury.

Back by B488 for $\frac{1}{4}$ mile, then left on B489, passing below Ivinghoe Beacon to the Traveller's Rest Inn (2$\frac{1}{2}$ miles) from which Edlesborough lies 1 mile left on B486.

Edlesborough, on an isolated chalk knoll facing the Chilterns, has a 13th-15th century Church with a 15th century pulpit which has a finely-carved canopy.

B489 on from the Traveller's Rest to the Plough Inn (1 mile), then B4506 (right) and B4540 (left), ascending the escarpment to Whipsnade Zoo (1$\frac{1}{2}$ miles).

Whipsnade Zoo (admission from 10 a.m., weekdays to 7 or dusk, Sundays and Bank Holidays to 7.30 or dusk), on the Chiltern plateau, occupies a large open space administered by the Zoological Society of London. It was founded in 1931 by Sir Peter Chalmers Mitchell with the object of allowing wild animals from all over the world to live in uncaged freedom in paddocks and of preserving rare animals that are in danger of becoming extinct. Carved in the face of the escarpment is a ' white lion ' 200 yards long. To the north of the green at Whipsnade village (see below) is a ' Tree Cathedral ' with a variety of species.

B4540 on through Whipsnade ($\frac{1}{2}$ mile), then by an unclassified road in $\frac{1}{2}$ mile more, passing through Studham (2 miles farther) to Clement's End ($\frac{1}{2}$ mile), then by another unclassified road (forking right) over B486 (which leads left direct to Water End and Hemel Hempstead) and ascending across Hudnall Common to Little Gaddesden (2$\frac{1}{2}$ miles).

Little Gaddesden is an attractive village on a Chiltern ridge, with 15th century and later houses bordering a long green, among them the Elizabethan Manor House (admission Easter-September, Sundays and Bank Holidays, 2 to 6; also Wednesdays in July and August), which has contemporary wall paintings and early keyboard instruments. The much-rebuilt Church, $\frac{1}{2}$ mile north of this, contains 17th-19th century monuments of the Earls and Countesses of Bridgwater, who lived from 1604 at Ashridge (admission to gardens, April-September, Saturdays, Sundays and Bank Holidays, 2 to 6, to the house on a few days only), a huge Gothic mansion rebuilt in 1808-14 by James Wyatt and his nephew, Sir Jeffry Wyatville. Now housing the Ashridge Management College, founded in 1959 to serve the needs of industry and business, it stands in grounds landscaped by ' Capability ' Brown and Humphry Repton. Part of the beautifully-wooded park is included in the Ashridge Estate of the National Trust, which extends as an open deer-park to Aldbury Common and Ivinghoe Beacon, and south to Berkhamsted Common.

Unclassified road south along the ridge to Nettleden (2 miles), then left into the Gade valley at Water End (1 mile), then by B486 (right) and an unclassified road (left) to Piccotts End (1$\frac{1}{2}$ miles).

Piccotts End is a hamlet with a row of cottages concealing a hall house (admission daily, 10 to 6 or 7.30) which has 14th century wall paintings of religious scenes, discovered in 1953.

Unclassified road on to Hemel Hempstead (1 mile).

Hemel Hempstead is a market town in the Gade valley, with a delightful High Street which has many 18th century houses. The large Church has original Norman work in the rib-vaulted chancel, the nave and the crossing tower, which has a later leaden spire, 200 feet high. It overlooks Gadebridge Park, in which (beyond B486) a large Roman villa is being excavated. To the south is the nucleus of the New Town developed since 1947 as a ·' satellite ' to London. The town centre, with the Town Hall and the fine Pavilion (for concerts, etc.), both built in 1966, is pleasantly laid out with water gardens and sculpture. The quickest route to London follows A414 and A4147 left to join the M1 Motorway.

A4146 on to Apsley (1 mile), then A41 (left; often busy) to Kings Langley (2 miles).

Kings Langley, in the Gade valley, is a mainly residential village with some old houses and a 15th century Church containing a fine tomb-chest perhaps intended for Richard II, who was first buried here. It became the burial-place of his uncle, Edmund de Langley, Duke of York, the son of Edward III.

A41 on via Hunton Bridge (Abbots Langley; $1\frac{1}{2}$ miles), then A411 (right) in 1 mile more to Watford (2 miles). [A41 (the Watford By-Pass), to the left at the fork, crosses the M1, a much quicker route to London.]

Watford is a busy market and manufacturing town on the Colne, with a much-restored 13th and 15th century Parish Church (near the High Street), which has interesting brasses and monuments.

A411 on to Bushey (2 miles), then A4140 (right) is 1 mile more to Bushey Heath (1 mile), then A409 (right) through Harrow Weald to Harrow Station (3 miles), beyond which A4005 ascends (right) to Harrow-on-the-Hill ($1\frac{1}{2}$ miles).

Harrow-on-the-Hill stands on the top of a hill rising conspicuously above the plain. It has pleasant 18th century houses, but is most famous for Harrow School, one of the foremost public schools in England, founded in 1571 by John Lyon, a yeoman of the parish, and granted a charter by Elizabeth I. The Old Schools, enlarged in 1820, include the ' Fourth Form Room ' (1611), with panels carved with the names of famous pupils. The restored 12th-15th century Parish Church has good brasses, including that of John Lyon, and a distinctive spire. It stands in a churchyard that affords an extensive view over north-west London.

A4005 on to Sudbury (2 miles), then A404 (Harrow Road; left) through Wembley and across the North Circular Road (2 miles more), then on via Harlesden and Kensal Green to reach Edgware Road (A5) over $\frac{1}{2}$ mile short of Marble Arch ($5\frac{1}{2}$ miles).

Letchworth Ba...

A505 A6141

Hitchin

A600

A602
Stevenage

St.Paul's Walden

Whitwell

A1(M)

Knebworth House

B651

Kimpton

Knebworth

B197

Ayot St. Lawrence

A6115

A600 **Welwyn**

Wheathampstead

A1 **Welwyn Garden City**

A414 **Hertford**

B651 **Hertingfordbury**

A602

Hertford Heath

Gorhambury

B556 **Hatfield**

Hoddesdon

St.Albans

Verulamium

Broxbourne

A1 A10

London Colney

A6

A1010

Salisbury Hall

Cheshunt

South Mimms

Waltham Cross
A105

M1

A1

A10

A406

Mill Hill

A1

Finchley

M1

A41

Hendon

A598

Golders Green

A406

Tour 10
96 miles

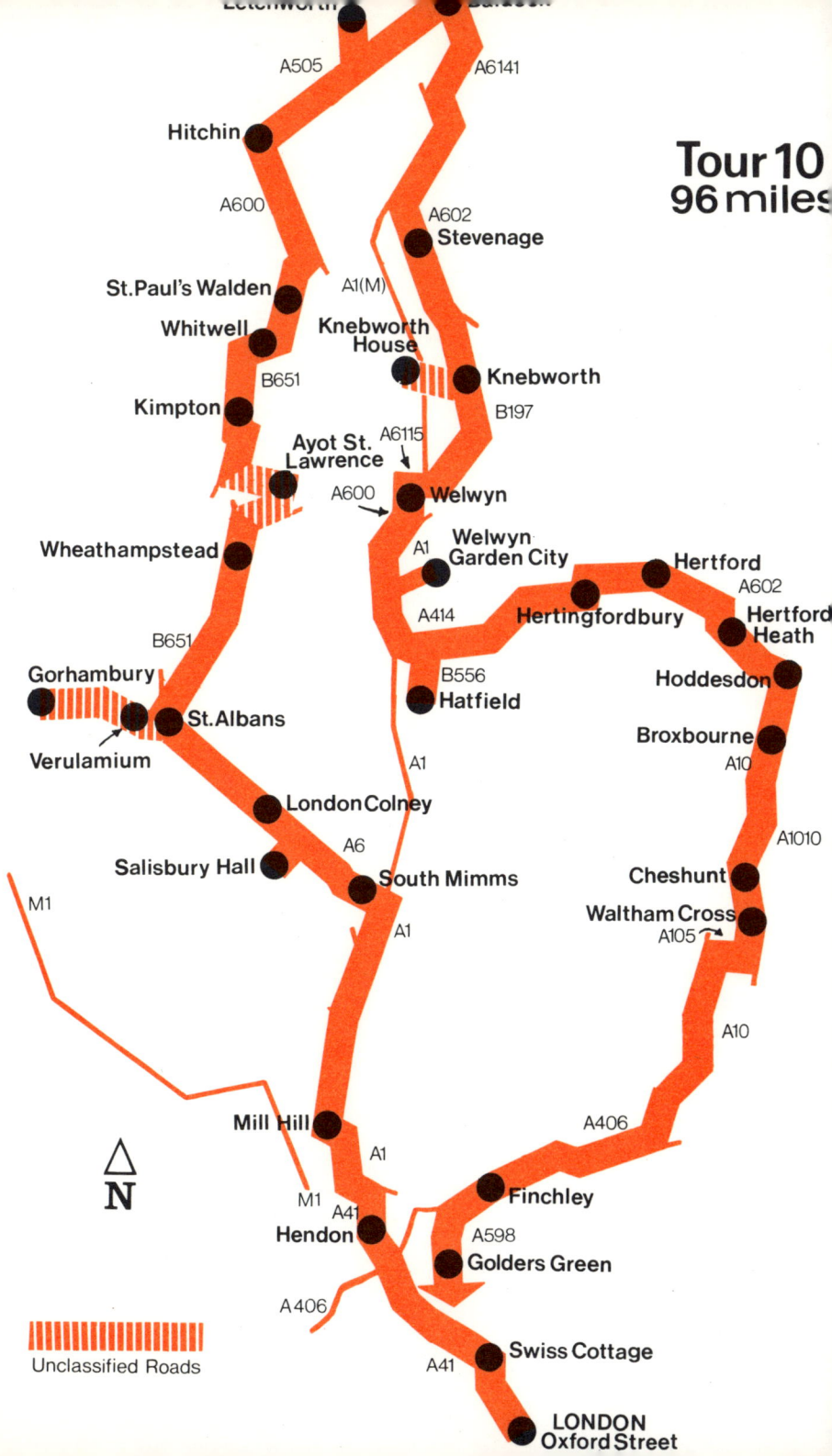

||||| **Unclassified Roads**

N

Swiss Cottage

A41

LONDON Oxford Street

10. St. Albans, the Hertfordshire Uplands and the Lea Valley

This tour covers the Hertfordshire uplands, the " hearty, homely, loving Hertfordshire " of Charles Lamb. It takes in the fascinating old cathedral city of St. Albans and the near-by Roman remains of Verulamium; the old towns of Hitchin, Baldock and Hertford, and the varied ' new towns ' of Letchworth (the first garden city), Stevenage and Welwyn Garden City; interesting villages such as Ayot St. Lawrence, the home of Bernard Shaw; St. Paul's Walden, with the early home of the Queen Mother; and great houses like Gorhambury and the Elizabethan Hatfield House. The return is made through the valley of the Lea or Lee.

From London (Oxford Street) by Portman Street and Gloucester Place, then by Park Road and A41 via St. John's Wood, Swiss Cottage, Hampstead (Finchley Road) and Hendon Way, crossing the North Circular Road to Hendon (6½ miles). A41 (Watford Way) on to join A1 in 1 mile, then via Mill Hill and Barnet Way to South Mimms (6½ miles); then A6 (left) to London Colney (4½ miles), passing the approach to Salisbury Hall.

South Mimms has an interesting Church with features of the 13th-16th centuries. Salisbury Hall (admission Easter-September, Sundays, 2 to 6; also Thursdays from July; Bank Holidays 10.30 to 5.30) is a moated 16th-17th century manor house.

A6 on to St. Albans (3½ miles).

St. Albans is a market and residential town on a hill above the Ver, with many old houses in its interesting streets. It first grew up round a Benedictine abbey founded in the 8th century by Offa, King of Mercia. The Cathedral, originally the abbey church, has a massive Norman tower constructed of Roman bricks and the longest medieval nave in Europe. The transepts and part of the nave are Norman work, the presbytery is mostly of the 13th century and the Lady Chapel at the east end is of the 14th century, but the west front was recast after 1879 by Lord Grimthorpe at his own expense. The cathedral has interesting wall paintings and monuments, and behind the altar screen is the restored shrine of St. Alban, a Roman soldier, the first Christian martyr in England, who was beheaded here in about A.D. 303. To the west of the cathedral is the great 14th century Abbey Gatehouse, now part of St. Albans School, traditionally founded before the Norman Conquest. The lane through the gate descends to the Fighting Cocks Inn, a quaint octagonal timber-framed building, near the small river Ver. The 15th century Curfew Tower, facing the High Street, is one of the only two in England. From it, the narrow French Row, preserving its medieval appearance, leads north to the Market Place and the Town Hall of 1831, from which the tree-lined St. Peter's Street goes on past the entrance to the fine Civic Centre, completed in 1967, to St. Peter's, a 16th century

59

church with a Victorian exterior. In Hatfield Road, to the east, is the City Museum (admission weekdays, 10 to 4 or 5.30), which has exhibits of local history, a fine collection of tools, and a reconstruction of a village workshop. George Street and Fishpool Street, with many delightful old houses, descend from the High Street towards St. Michael's Church, which has Saxon walls but was over-restored by Lord Grimthorpe. It contains a monument to Francis Bacon, the statesman and philosopher, who died in 1626 and is probably buried here. Near by, in a pleasant park, is the site of the large Roman city of Verulamium, established soon after the conquest of A.D. 43. The remains include parts of the city wall with the south-east gate and a large mosaic floor over a hypocaust. The Verulamium Museum (admission 10 to 4 or 5.30; Sundays from 2) contains other fine floors and an excellent collection of pottery, glassware, metalwork and wall paintings. On the other side of the by-pass road is the Roman Theatre, built in A.D. 140 and the only one of its kind in Britain. The drive passing it goes on to Gorhambury (admission May-September, Thursdays and Fridays, 2 to 6; also the second Saturdays and Sundays in May, June and September), a classical mansion built in 1777-84 by Sir Robert Taylor, with numerous family and other portraits and busts of Sir Nicholas Bacon and his son, Francis Bacon.

A6 and B651 (right; reached also from the by-pass) north from St. Albans to Sandridge and thence to Wheathampstead (4½ miles).

Wheathampstead is a large village on the upper course of the Lea, with an interesting 13th-14th century Church. The Devil's Dyke, ½ mile east and reached by B653, is part of the earthwork that enclosed the Belgic capital of the Catuvellauni.

B651 on over the river, then by an unclassified road right, with a left fork in 1 mile, to Ayot St. Lawrence (2½ miles).

Ayot St. Lawrence is a secluded village among the leafy Hertford-shire lanes. Shaw's Corner (admission Tuesday-Sunday and Bank Holiday Mondays, 11 to 1 and 2 to 6 or dusk; closed on Bank Holiday Tuesdays), the home of George Bernard Shaw from 1906 until his death in 1950, still remains very much as it was in his lifetime, with many interesting mementoes. The 18th century ' Grecian ' Church stands in the grounds of Ayot House, which contains the Lullingstone Silk Farm (admission April-September, daily until 5.45).

Unclassified road west from Shaw's Corner for 1½ miles, then B651 (right) to Kimpton (1 mile more) and thence via Whitwell to St. Paul's Walden (3 miles farther).

St. Paul's Walden is a hamlet with a 14th-15th century Church which has a Gothick chancel remodelled in the 18th century. It stands at the north end of the park of St. Paul's Walden Bury, an 18th-19th century house, the home of the Bowes-Lyon family, where Queen Elizabeth, the Queen Mother, was born in 1900.

B651 on for 2 miles, then A600 (right) to Hitchin (3 miles more).

Hitchin is an attractive market town with rose and herb gardens and numerous 16th-18th century houses, mostly around the Market Place. The large and interesting Parish Church has 14th century nave arcades, but is mainly of the 15th century and has many 15th-16th century brasses.

A505 east to Letchworth (3 miles), which lies north of the road.

Letchworth, the first 'garden city' in the world, was founded in 1903 under the inspiration of Ebenezer Howard and laid out by Barry Parker and Sir Raymond Unwin. The principal buildings, all around The Broadway, include the Museum and Art Gallery (admission weekdays, except Bank Holidays, 10 to 5), which has good local history and natural history collections.

A505 on east to Baldock (2 miles).

Baldock, below the escarpment of the chalklands that extend the Chilterns, is an old coaching town on the old Great North Road, with wide streets and many 18th century houses.

A6141 (formerly A1) south for 2 miles, then A1(M) left for $2\frac{1}{2}$ miles and A602 (left again) to Stevenage ($1\frac{1}{2}$ miles).

Stevenage is another old coaching town, with a broad High Street. To the east and south-east of this a New Town, designated in 1946 and the first of its kind in England, is growing up.

A602 on for 2 miles, then B197 (right) to Knebworth ($1\frac{1}{2}$ miles).

Knebworth consists of a newer part, built round the station and the main road, and Old Knebworth, over a mile west up the hill. Here is the entrance to Knebworth House (admission May-September, Saturdays, Sundays and Bank Holidays, 2.30 to 5.30), the ancestral seat of the Lytton family, a Tudor mansion almost completely recast in the Gothic style after 1811. The banqueting hall has family portraits and 17th century woodwork. The much restored Church, in the park, contains pretentious 18th century monuments of the Lyttons.

B197 on for $2\frac{1}{2}$ miles, then A6115 on to Welwyn ($\frac{1}{2}$ mile), beyond which it passes west of Welwyn Garden City, reached by B190.

Welwyn is a small town on the Maran or Mimram, with attractive old houses and inns. Welwyn Garden City, founded in 1920 as a 'satellite' town to London, was laid out by Louis de Soissons and A. W. Kenyon on the lines of Letchworth, with regular streets and squares. In 1948 it was designated a New Town.

A600 (left) and A1 (right) for $4\frac{1}{2}$ miles from Welwyn, then A414 (left) for $\frac{3}{4}$ mile and B556 (right) to Hatfield ($\frac{3}{4}$ mile more).

Hatfield is an old market town with charming 18th century houses in Fore Street, which ascends to the Parish Church, partly of the 13th and 15th centuries but with a nave of 1872. The Salisbury Chapel, of 1618, has fine 18th century Flemish ironwork gates and the elaborate monument of Robert Cecil, 1st Earl of Salisbury, son of the Elizabethan statesman, Lord Burghley. An extension

of Hatfield to the west and south-west was designated a New Town in 1948. To the east, in a delightful park, is Hatfield House (admission Easter Saturday and Sunday, and weekdays to the end of April; then Tuesday-Sunday and Bank Holidays to early October; 12 to 5, Sundays, 2.30 to 5.30), the stately Jacobean mansion of the Earls and Marquesses of Salisbury, built in 1607-11 by Robert Lyminge. The state rooms, partly altered by the 3rd Marquess, the Prime Minister, who died in 1903, include the Marble Hall, with a fine screen and gallery and portraits of Elizabeth I, and the Long Gallery, which has relics of the queen. In the beautiful gardens is the wing of the Bishop's Palace, built by Cardinal Morton in 1497.

B556 back for $\frac{3}{4}$ mile, then A414 (right), crossing the Lea, to Hertingfordbury ($4\frac{3}{4}$ miles).

Hertingfordbury, in the wooded valley of the Mimram, is an attractive village with a restored Church, partly of the 13th century.

A414 on to Hertford ($1\frac{1}{2}$ miles).

Hertford, well situated in the valley of the Lea, is a delightful county town with important corn and cattle markets. Its many old buildings include the Shire Hall (by James Adam, 1769) in Fore Street, and the 15th century timber-framed Old Verger's House, in St. Andrew Street. The Museum (admission daily, 10 to 1 and 2 to 4 or 5), in Bull Plain, contains local antiquities and ' bygones '. Of the Castle there survives a Norman motte or mound, a length of curtain wall, and the much-altered 16th century gatehouse. In the Ware road (A414; see below) is Christ's Hospital School for Girls, founded in London in 1553 and moved here in 1778 to new buildings beside the boys' school. When the boys moved to Sussex, in 1902, their school was taken over and rebuilt for the girls.

A414 east and A602 (right) to Hoddesdon ($4\frac{1}{2}$ miles), then A10 (right) to Broxbourne (1 mile).

Hoddesdon is a market town west of the Lea where it is joined by the Stort. Broxbourne, which adjoins it on the south, has a complete church in the Perpendicular style.

A10 on for $1\frac{1}{2}$ miles, then A1010 (left) to Cheshunt (2 miles more) and thence to Waltham Cross (1 mile).

Waltham Cross (like Cheshunt) is a residential town in the Lea valley, along which are numerous market gardens. The well-restored Eleanor Cross is one of the three surviving of the thirteen erected by Edward I to mark the resting places of the cortege of his queen on its journey (in 1290) to Westminster Abbey.

A1010 on from Waltham Cross for $\frac{1}{2}$ mile, then A105 (right) for 1 mile to rejoin A10 (left) for 5 miles; then A406 (North Circular Road; right) through Finchley for $5\frac{1}{2}$ miles and A598 (left) via Golders Green ($1\frac{1}{2}$ miles), $\frac{1}{2}$ mile beyond which the tour meets the outgoing route. The centre of London (Oxford Street), 4 miles farther, is reached by Park Road, Baker Street and Orchard Street.

62

Index of Places

Special Free Tickets for readers of

Letts Motor Tour Guides   VALUE **12/6**

THAMES VALLEY

Mapledurham House, Mapledurham

SEE PAGE 22

This ticket issued by kind permission of

J. J. Eyston, Esq.

Letts Motor Tour Guides

Easter Sun. to Sept. 28 Sats. and Suns. 2.30-5.30. Bank Holidays only Sats., Suns., Mons. and Tues.)

VALUE **3/6**

Valid only when accompanied by one or more paying visitors

Nether Winchenden House, Aylesbury

SEE PAGE 39

This ticket issued by kind permission of

J. G. C. Spencer Bernard, Esq.

Letts Motor Tour Guides

May to Aug.—Thurs. 2-6; also Easter Mon., Spring and late Summer Bank Holidays 2-6

VALUE **3/-**

Valid only when accompanied by one or more paying visitors

Milton Manor House, Abingdon

SEE PAGE 28

This ticket issued by kind permission of

Surgeon Capt. and Mrs E. J. Mockler

Letts Motor Tour Guides

May 3 to Sept. 28—Sats. and Suns; also Spring and late Summer Bank Holidays 2.30-6

VALUE **3/6**

Valid only when accompanied by one or more paying visitors

Ditchley Park Enstone

SEE PAGE 34

This ticket issued by kind permission of

The Ditchley Foundation

Letts Motor Tour Guides

July 21 to Aug. 1 only 2-5

VALUE **2/6**

Valid only when accompanied by one or more paying visitors